A CANCER
BATTLE PLAN
SOURCEBOOK

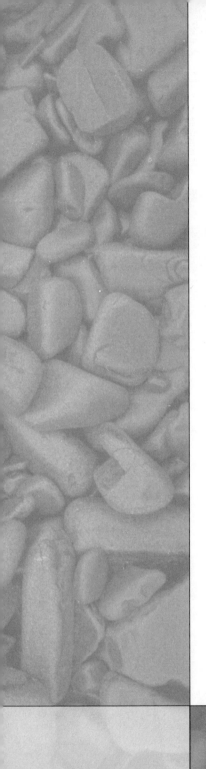

Also by Dave Frähm

A Cancer Battle Plan (with Anne Frähm)

Healthy Habits (with Anne Frähm)

Reclaim Your Health (with Anne Frähm)

A CANCER BATTLE PLAN SOURCEBOOK

A Step-by-Step Health Program to Give Your Body a Fighting Chance

DAVE FRÄHM

Jeremy P. Tarcher/Putnam
a member of
Penguin Putnam Inc.
New York

Most Tarcher/Putnam books are available at special quantity discounts for bulk purchase for sales promotions, premiums, fund-raising, and educational needs. Special books or book excerpts also can be created to fit specific needs. For details, write Putnam Special Markets, 375 Hudson Street, New York, NY 10014.

Jeremy P. Tarcher/Putnam
A member of
Penguin Putnam Inc.
375 Hudson Street
New York, NY 10014
www.penguinputnam.com

Library of Congress Cataloging-in-Publication Data

Frähm, David J.
    A cancer battle plan sourcebook : a step-by-step health
program to give your body a fighting chance / David Frähm.
        p.   cm.
    Includes bibliographical references.
    ISBN 1-58542-002-6
    1. Cancer—Alternative treatment.   2. Naturopathy.   I. Title.
    RC271.A62 F73   2000   99-049522 CIP
    616.99'406—dc21

Printed in the United States of America

10 9 8 7 6 5 4 3 2 1

This book is printed on acid-free paper. ∞

Book design by Tanya Maiboroda

ACKNOWLEDGMENTS

I THANK MY WIFE, Anne Frähm. It was her sense of calling from God, and her purpose and passion within that calling, that brought us to the ministry of helping people better their health. Her legacy lives in the gratitude felt by those who have benefited from her work.

I thank Trisha Anderson, Camice Hernandez, Sharon Brechtl, and Frank Myers—four key pillars on whom the infrastructure of Health*Quarters* Ministries rests. Without them, this book could not have been written. Not just co-laborers, but true friends. In every way, you have my heart.

Thank you to all who over the years have attended one of our Lodge sessions or visited my office as clients. Your confidence in my services has allowed me to hone my skills in reading what the body is asking for.

To publisher Joel Fotinos of Tarcher/Putnam, thanks for believing. And to David Groff, thanks for your expert editing.

And finally, thank you to God who gave me the love of words and brought me to the ministry of health—a marriage made in heaven.

To Anne Elizabeth Frähm
A life well lived

CONTENTS

PREFACE

I'M HAPPY THAT you've picked up this sourcebook, meant as a follow-up to *A Cancer Battle Plan*. It includes the principles of detoxification and nutrition covered in that book, yet expands and goes beyond.

Most of what's presented here is what I teach participants in the 11-day Health*Quarters* Ministries Lodge programs (see appendix A). My primary goal is to help you regain a sense of control over your own body and its health. Of all the people in the world who ought to know the most about how to take care of your body, it ought to be you.

As you work your way through *A Cancer Battle Plan Sourcebook,* if you have questions, please don't hesitate to contact Health*Quarters* Ministries at (719) 593-8694 or interact with us through our Website at www. healthquarters.org. (For more information, see appendix A.) We're here to serve. And if you're ever in the Colorado Springs area, stop in and see us at 955 Garden of the Gods Road.

Dave Frähm, N.D., CNC, CNHP

A FIGHTING

CHANCE

1

YOUR BODY
IS THE HERO

THE HUMAN BODY was designed by God to be naturally self-healing and self-protective. It is the healer. Your body is ever and always moving toward self-protection and repair. Cut yourself, and you'll soon find a clot, then a scab—a healing in process. Break a bone, and the body will lay down mineral deposits to heal it. Come under the attack of a virus, and the body will send its police force (white blood cells) to arrest and purge the invader.

A truth about your body of which you may be unaware, though, is that you have as many as ten thousand cancer cells floating around inside. You, me, the neighbor next door have all got cancer cells. Here again, though, is part of the marvelous design of our bodies. That force that goes after a virus is also designed to seek out and destroy mutant cells we call cancer. No problem.

TEAMWORK IN ACTION

The body you inhabit is a synergistic city of cells—one hundred trillion of them. Each has an important individual role to play and in so doing supports the working of the whole. Taking a tour inside yourself, you'd find

**Frähm's Principle
of Good Health**

In all matters of health
and healing, the body is
the hero.

**Frähm's Principle
of Good Health**

When it comes to most
matters of health, we
reap what we sow. Each
of us needs to learn to
make choices that give
the protective and heal-
ing powers in our bodies
a fighting chance.

teams of cellular employees manning industries and systems, keeping your cellular city running smoothly.

You'd find billions working the communications infrastructure that keeps every cell in touch with the command and control center—your brain. Other huge teams would be employed in food warehouses, water purification systems, energy production plants, heating and ventilation systems, and the learning center.

A poet-king once pondered the unique gift we've all been given: "You [God] made all the delicate, inner parts of my body, and knit them together in my mother's womb. Thank you for making me so wonderfully complex! It is amazing to think about. Your workmanship is marvelous—and how well I know it."[1]

WHAT'S THE DEAL WITH CANCER?

I see that question more often than I hear it. I see it in the eyes of folks that come to me looking for help and hope. I teach at a Lodge where people come from all over the country to learn how to take better care of their bodies. Their eyes often ask, "If my body's so wonderful, so self-healing, then why am I so sick?"

The fundamental truth about many of the degenerative diseases that now plague America (cancer, heart/circulatory disease, stroke, diabetes, arthritis, fibromyalgia, chronic fatigue syndrome, osteoporosis, and others) is that we have brought them upon ourselves, even if mostly out of ignorance.

We simply do not comprehend the care and feeding of the human body. As a result, our collective health is suffering. The American Medical Association and the World Health Organization confirm that we are now in the midst of the worst epidemic of chronic and degenerative disease that the world has ever known.

COMMITTING YOURSELF TO THE CAUSE

This book is about just that—learning how to give your body a fighting chance against cancer in a world where winning back or simply maintaining good health takes work, commitment, common sense, working knowledge, and support.

By reading the opening pages of this book, you're showing promise in that direction. Reading, though, will not be enough. Success at keeping or rebuilding health can only be attained if you are willing to make changes and practice self-discipline.

It's your body. You're in charge of the war effort. Everyone else is hired help. Are you ready to do what it takes to win back and cultivate good health? Sign your name and write the date here. Let this be your pledge to yourself and your long-term health.

Name _____

Date _____

2

LIGHTEN YOUR TOXIC LOAD

A MAN DROVE through the mountains one day, stopping now and then to load rocks into his trunk. With each new rock, his car got slower and slower. It sagged lower and lower, too.

He stopped to toss in yet another rock, when all of a sudden—BAMMM!—his car's suspension gave way. The gas tank slammed to the pavement, sparks flew, gasoline ignited. The authorities arrived on the scene only to find that nothing remained of the man and his car but twisted metal and smoking ashes.

What could the man have done to save his car, and what could he have done to prevent his death? That is the fundamental question that often stands between good health and bad—between disease-free living and sickness.

Answering that question is the foundation for all that we do and teach at Health*Quarters* Lodge, where people come to learn and to put into practice diet and lifestyle changes that will give their body a fighting chance in the battle against cancer. (See appendix A.)

OVERCOMING THE "DRAGS AND SAGS"

Common sense dictates that our unfortunate man's first step would have been to quit adding to the pile of rocks already in his trunk. Anyone could see there was a definite "cause and effect" relationship between the rocks he was carrying and the troubles he was experiencing.

In that light, his second step would have been equally as obvious— clean out the rocks already there. It would've made complete sense, too, given his tendency to want to pick up rocks, that at some point he should have invested time and money in strengthening his suspension system.

Our bodies are like that car. You and I go through life accumulating various kinds of "rocks" (stressors), knowingly or not, that place a growing burden on the body's ability to function normally. These are "toxic" stressors, for anything that the body doesn't require in order to stay healthy and that taxes the body to deal with can rightly be called a toxin.

Along the road through life the total load of toxic stressors can become too much. Physical breakdown occurs. A major health crisis sets in—cancer and other degenerative conditions like heart attack, stroke, diabetes, Alzheimer's, multiple sclerosis, chronic fatigue syndrome, arthritis, allergies, and many, many other such crises. They are conditions in which the normal functionings of the body's various systems, working together to fight disease and produce health, have become compromised. There are too many "rocks" in the trunk.

As I mentioned in chapter 1, scientists tell us that each of us has as many as ten thousand cancer cells floating around in our body at all times. A body that is in "homeostasis," when every organ is performing its duty, destroys them quite effectively. However, when homeostasis is disrupted by "toxic stressor overload," freelancing cancer cells have a chance to get organized into mobs. Tumors result. This same disruption of homeostasis is the culprit behind all types of degenerative conditions. It only makes sense that anyone fighting or wishing to avoid cancer or any other sort of degenerative condition would want to make three things a foundational part of a personal battle plan, regardless of whatever else he or she did:

1. Avoid further contact with toxic stressors.

2. Clean out the toxic buildup already there.

3. Restore and strengthen the body's own protecting and healing powers.

Frähm's Principle of Good Health

There really is only one degenerative disease of the human body—toxic overload. Everything else is a symptom.

Frähm's Principle of Good Health
The only cure for cancer is the body itself.

THERE IS HOPE DOWN THIS ROAD

If you haven't already read *A Cancer Battle Plan,* let me suggest that you do so. In it you'll find our story of what we did originally to win back Anne's (my wife's) health from so-called terminal breast cancer (stage 4—the worst). Not knowing at first that there were other ways to help combat cancer, we headed down the path most familiar—surgery, radiation, chemotherapy, hormone therapy, even a bone marrow transplant.

These radical and highly invasive therapies did at first help to reduce the cancer load on Anne's system. When they failed to completely eradicate the disease, however, the medical community set us adrift. It took a friend to suggest that we consult with a nutritionist who set us on a path toward health and healing. What we discovered was that although the "big three" in the typical cancer-fighting toolbox can be potentially helpful tools, they serve only to slow down the disease process. They actually heal nothing.

Surgery, radiation, and chemotherapy are like a wolf chewing off its leg to get out of a trap. Its immediate problem may have been temporarily resolved, but long-term survival is in serious doubt.

The nutritionist we sought out put Anne on a strict program of diet and internal cleansing designed to "detoxify" her liver and colon, plus flood her system with nutrients to help rebuild and strengthen her immune system. As a result, there was a dramatic shift in her health status.

The cancer was gone.

Anne regained her health through rebuilding her whole system. Our phone rang day and night. Fellow cancer warriors, desperate for hope and help, wanted to know what she'd done. It became apparent that if we were to get any sleep, a book would need to be written. Thus, *A Cancer Battle Plan* was born.

Others began calling—people who didn't have cancer and wanted to keep it that way. "What can we do to stay healthy?" was their question. We responded with our second book, *Healthy Habits: 20 Simple Ways to Improve Your Health.* Many "home schoolers" now use this book as their text for teaching children about nutrition.

Still other people called. "I've read *A Cancer Battle Plan* and see that this detoxification and immune system–rebuilding approach worked for Anne, but has it worked for anyone else?"

We responded with yet another book, *Reclaim Your Health: Nutritional*

Strategies for Conquering Chronic Ailments. In it we told fifty success stories of people who had used the "detox and rebuild" model of *A Cancer Battle Plan* to win back their health from a variety of health challenges, including MS, diabetes, arthritis, allergies, chronic fatigue syndrome, mental illness, AIDS, and more.

BUT YOU GOTTA UNLOAD ALL THE BIG ROCKS

Having said all that, it's important that you know that Anne has left this world. Anne was plagued by troublesome symptoms for the last months of her life. Blood tests revealed an increase of cancer cells to which she'd responded by redoubling her efforts at juice fasting, colon cleansing, and the 80/20 diet (all things covered in this book). We began seeing a holistic-minded physician, who traced the source of the development of a tumor in Anne's ovaries to infection in the jawbone beneath a specific tooth. A "biologically trained" dentist was enlisted to drill a hole in the bone and flood the infected area with homeopathic remedies to kill the offending bacteria. The ovarian tumor went away.

That experience taught us how devastating cavitations—infections in the jawbone—can be to one's health. Only late in the game were three more discovered and oral surgeries performed to open them up to clean out the toxic bacteria holed up there. The bacteria had a direct link to the bloodstream via bone tissue.

There were other "rocks." Perhaps the biggest one that we were unable to address effectively was the iron poisoning Anne had in her body as the result of having received over 150 blood transfusions during the failed bone marrow transplant. With any transfusion of blood, you get a whopping dose of the donor's iron. Being in chemical menopause, Anne was unable to flush excess iron from her system through normal means.

We tried chelation therapy, in most cases a valuable tool but in Anne's case discouraging. Not only is excess iron a huge manufacturer of what are called free radicals, which wound tissues and are the genesis of disease processes, but iron is also "food" for bacteria like that found in abundance in Anne's jawbone. The massive iron stores in her body were a feeding trough.

White blood cells, our protective agents against both bacteria and cancer cells, are attracted to the iron in bacteria, thus making contact and killing them. However, when there are excess stores of iron, white blood cells attach themselves to this excess iron and are thus unavailable for our protection. Free radicals do their damage to cells and tissues. Bacteria thrive. Cancer cells multiply and form tumors. Parasites have a heyday.

We were doing all that we knew to do to "detox" Anne's system, but sometimes you don't know what you're dealing with or what to do about it before great damage has already been done. Ignorance doesn't protect us from reality.

Until late in the game we knew nothing about the cavitations. Had we been fully aware of the dramatic importance of these lingering challenges to her immune system, even though the cancer had been conquered years before, I'm confident Anne would still be hard at work beside me, helping others.

WHY THIS BOOK?

I want you to learn from our successes and avoid our failures. *A Cancer Battle Plan* was our story of success during our first go-around with the disease. Originally given just a handful of months to live, Anne stretched that out to nearly 10 years. Colon and liver detoxing, plus dietary changes and mega-supplements, were immensely important.

The iron poisoning that was part of her eventual demise was a "rock" that came by way of the original cancer treatment we'd chosen. You need to know that. You also need to know about cavitations and other dental stressors, something we didn't cover in depth in *A Cancer Battle Plan*.

A Cancer Battle Plan was more a story of one woman's successful experience than a plan to be followed. In the years that have followed, people have asked again and again for step-by-step help in the "detox and rebuild" process. This manual is my attempt to address that need.

In chapters 3–8 my focus is to inform you about the "rocks." It won't be unusual to feel a bit overwhelmed at first. There are a lot of things that add to the load of stress that the average American body is dealing with.

The focus of chapters 9–18 is to give you practical tools to help you "unload" or detoxify your body. All these chapters are important, but none is more critical than chapter 18, "Juice Fasting and Colon/Liver Cleansing." This is the focal point of any serious program of detoxification. Many of the other "unloading" tools mentioned fit into the context of a juice fast. You'll find sample plans at the end of chapter 18.

Chapters 19–27 present tools for stimulating and strengthening your body's healing powers. All are important, but one stands out as crucial—in chapter 19, the 80/20 diet. The chemistry you feed your body on a daily basis is of utmost importance to your ability to regain and maintain health.

In chapters 28–35, I introduce you to tools you can use to help identify how your body is doing. The three tools I consider most crucial are muscle response testing, iridology, and the AMAS blood test.

Finally, in chapter 36, I share with you the characteristics I've observed in people who do well at winning back their health using the kind of information provided in this book.

Remember that good health takes work!

THE ROCKS

3

TOXIC DIET

The Eight Self-Inflicted

Wounds of the Standard

American Diet

THERE ARE AT LEAST EIGHT aspects of the standard American diet (S.A.D.) that qualify as self-inflicted wounds that can, and do, contribute to the development of cancer and other degenerative diseases in the human body.

- Too much protein
- Too much fat
- Too much sugar
- Too much salt
- Too much caffeine
- Too many chemicals
- Too many refined foods
- Too many cooked foods

TOO MUCH PROTEIN

Protein is the second most plentiful substance in the human body (after water), making up roughly one-fifth of our total weight (or about three-quarters of the solid parts of the body). It is the key constituent of every cell and body fluid, with the exception of bile and urine.

Protein in the diet is used by the body

- To form, maintain, and repair all bodily tissues

- To build enzymes and hormones that run bodily systems and functions

- To build hemoglobin and other blood proteins that deliver nutrients, regulate water balance and osmotic pressure (the equality of pressure between fluids on either side of the cell wall), and help maintain acid-alkaline balance

- To build antibodies that fight infection and disease

- And in diets where not enough carbohydrates and fats are consumed to satisfy energy needs, the body will burn dietary proteins to meet its energy needs, then protein tissues in the body—a reason why so many weight-loss diets are high protein/low carbohydrate and why they're so dangerous to long-term health.

Of all the major nutrients in the human diet, protein is the most discussed. The two key questions are always (1) How much does a body need? and (2) What are the best food sources?

How Much Does a Body Need?

The World Health Organization (WHO) has stated that the daily minimum requirement for protein in the human diet should be about 5 percent of calories consumed.

Take 5 percent of the 3,000 calories consumed on a typical day by an average American working man. It equals 150 calories. Dividing 150 by 4, since a gram of protein equals 4 calories, means that roughly 38 grams of protein are needed in the diet of the average man. Applying the same formula to the average American woman consuming 2,300 calories, that means 29 grams of protein.

John A. McDougall, M.D., from whose book *The McDougall Plan* these statistics have been taken, goes on to point out that "these minimum requirements provide for a large margin of safety that easily covers people who theoretically could have greater protein needs."[1]

There are many nutritionists and nutrition-minded medical doctors, including McDougall himself, who contend that the average body needs as little as 20 grams a day to keep its protein level at what it should be.

What Happens When You Consume Too Much?

While the body needs less than 40 grams a day, and according to some, closer to 20, the average American consumes somewhere between 105 and 120 grams of protein a day.

What happens in a body when it is fed too much protein? At least five things:

1. A weakening of the immune system
2. A weakening of the bones and joints
3. A weakening of the liver/gallbladder and fat metabolism
4. A weakening of the kidneys
5. A weakening of the colon

A weakening of the immune system

The pancreas plays a significant role in fighting cancer. It produces enzymes that help not only to break down and digest proteins in our foods but also to attack the protein coating around cancer cells, thus rendering them defenseless.

A healthy pancreas is able to produce a large enough enzymatic police force to accomplish both functions at once. However, many people lack such pancreatic power. For them, a diet high in animal products draws heavily on available enzymatic forces, diverting attention away from cancer cells.

A weakening of the bones and joints

There are two kinds of ash in the body as a result of the digestive process—either alkaline or acid. All animal products (meat, dairy, eggs, etc.) and things cooked (including most foods from the plant kingdom) burn down to an acid ash.

Your body makes acid as a natural by-product of cell life. It does not, however, make alkaline. The two combined—the high protein, acid-producing diet typical for most Americans plus the acid naturally produced by the body—make for acidic conditions.

In order to maintain health, the bloodstream must remain slightly alkaline. On a scale from 1 to 14, with 1 being acidic and 14 being alkaline (and 7 being neutral), the body works to keep the blood at 7.4. Should it drop to 7.2, the body dies.

In the wake of the standard American diet, the body is constantly on

↑Acid Condition
☐ ↑ protein
☐ typical Am. Diet
☐ natl body acid. production

MAKES ACID
NATURALLY as
BY product of
cell life

the look for alkalinizing help. It will draw calcium (an alkalinizing mineral) from its bones in order to alkalinize, and thus neutralize, the effects of too many acid-producing foods in the diet. Bone loss, otherwise known as osteoporosis, will be the long-term result. This free-floating calcium, before arriving at the kidneys for removal, may find a home in joints, resulting in arthritic conditions.

Wouldn't drinking milk help to supply the needed calcium? Dairy products burn to an acid ash in the human body. Milk consumption is not the solution to getting calcium to bones. It contributes to an acid condition, leading to bone loss.

A weakening of the liver/gallbladder and fat metabolism

Before the body takes calcium from bones, it will extract the alkalinizing sodium that holds cholesterol in liquid suspension in the gallbladder. With sodium gone, cholesterol hardens and gallstones form. This can lead to liver/gallbladder stress and poor fat metabolism, as the bile stored by the liver in the gallbladder is key to fat breakdown.

A weakening of the kidneys

When it comes to protein, more is not better. People eating a high protein diet most of their lives tend to end up with kidney problems. The body cannot store excess protein but must process and rid itself of what it cannot use each day. This is the job of the kidneys. Eating excessive amounts of protein on a daily basis puts a heavy burden on these vital organs.

Then, too, the free-floating calcium extracted from bones to help alkalinize the acids in the bloodstream produced by a high protein diet can also eventually cause additional problems for the kidneys—stones. With wounded, poorly functioning kidneys, toxic wastes they are meant to deal with get backed up into other organs and tissues. Diseases of all types can result.

A weakening of the colon

When we talk of too much protein in the American diet, we speak primarily of meat and dairy products, neither of which contains any fiber—none, zero, zip! Because the typical American consumes a lot of animal products and little fiber (which comes from plant sources), the transit time of animal protein slows, leading to putrifaction. Intestinal tissues can become wounded by this buildup of toxins. Colon cancers and related intestinal diseases can arise.

.   .   .

Where are you going to get your protein?

As you work your way through this manual, you'll see that I'm moving you toward a plant-based diet. The question you will be asking, or will have others ask you, is: Where are you going to get your protein on a vegetarian diet?

It's really quite simple. You make human protein from amino acids that come from the breakdown of foods you eat. Amino acids are the building blocks, the raw materials, from which human protein is manufactured.

You need roughly 23 different kinds of amino acids to make human protein. The way God has designed our bodies, we actually make 15 of these. That leaves us 8 short, which means they must come from our diets. Anything that must come from the outside because we don't make it on the inside is given the tag "essential." So there are 8 essential amino acids.

Can you get all 8 from plant sources? Yes!

Harvey Diamond, nutritionist and coauthor of *Fit for Life,* puts it this way: "If you eat any fruits, vegetables, grains, legumes, nuts, seeds or sprouts on a regular basis, you are receiving all the amino acids necessary for your body to build the protein it needs."[4]

When God designed man and put him in the original Garden, God knew what he was doing. You'll find me to be a big fan of the diet described in the first chapter of the book of Daniel in the Bible. Read it and see what you think.

Why is our country so concerned about getting enough protein?

Remember the famous Four Food Groups all schoolchildren were taught in grade school until recent times? Guess who came up with that "teaching" tool? No, it wasn't health-minded doctors and nutritionists who wanted to ensure good health. It was the American Dairy Association—a business entity with a vested interest in seeing to it that dairy products were sold. What better way than to indoctrinate young minds with the idea that without dairy every day, there would be something important missing from one's diet—namely, protein. Sure, they were kind enough to include meat as one of the food groups, which pleased the cattlemen and hog farmers, but isn't it interesting to note that dairy is listed in two of the four groups, making it appear to be the most important of all foods?

Uncle Sam liked this new marketing tool, and in 1956 the Department of Agriculture made the Four Food Groups the official health doctrine in public schools. From that point on, Americans were "taught" that if they didn't have the "protein foods" as part of every meal every day, they would be nutritionally lacking.

In more recent times doctors and nutritionists have shown that the Four Food Groups concept was a great deal of foolishness. Today school-teachers are teaching the Food Pyramid. Grains are the foundational food, and the next layer consists of fruits and vegetables. These foods provide all the body requires for health. All foods above this level on the pyramid are considered delicacies, not to be included in everyday fare.

Still, because of the marketing ploys of the meat and dairy industries, Americans worry if they're getting enough protein on their plates. Loyalty to a petrified opinion dies hard.

TOO MUCH FAT

We Americans live in the "fats lane." The average citizen's daily caloric intake is as much as 50 percent fat, most of it being the saturated kind found in animal products. As a result, our nation is plagued with circulatory diseases and cancer.

During both the Korean and Vietnam wars, autopsies were conducted on casualties on both sides. The bodies of American soldiers, averaging 18 to 20 years of age, already showed signs of hardening of the arteries due to a national diet high in saturated fats. The Asians showed no such degeneration. Their diet, of course, consists primarily of rice and veggies with a little fish—low in saturated fats.

In addition to circulatory diseases, it is a well-documented fact that when Asian women eat a Westernized diet, their rates of breast cancer sky-rocket. A multitude of studies clearly show the link between the high fat diet of the typical American and cancers of the colon and breast, second and third place, respectively, after lung cancer as the most commonly oc-curring cancers in our country.

In the December 1990 issue of the *New England Journal of Medicine,* results were given of the largest study ever conducted concerning the relationship between diet and colon cancer. The study had lasted six years and followed 88,751 women, 34 to 59 years of age. The results clearly revealed that as red meat and fat intake rose, so did the rates of colon cancer. The women eating the most animal fat could count on being twice as likely to develop colon cancer as those who ate the least amount.

Cancers of the gallbladder, pancreas, prostate, uterus, and ovaries have also been strongly correlated with high fat diets.

How does fat cause cancer?

Folks who study these things say that high fat diets cause cancer in at least a couple of ways.

- *Fat makes toxic wastes nastier.* Fat causes the liver to produce an abundance of bile acids to help break down the fat in the intestines. These acids stimulate and make more virulent cancer-causing toxic wastes already in the bowel as the result of other food and environmental sources.

- *Fat makes estrogens more numerous.* Fat in the intestinal tract gives rise to greater numbers of anaerobic bacteria, which in turn produce estrogens. An overabundance of estrogen (in relationship to progesterone, the other key female hormone) in the female body can lead to the production of tumors, most notably in the breast tissue. In males, excess estrogen (again, in relationship to progesterone) has the potential to cause prostrate cancer. (For more information about estrogens, progesterones, and hormone balancing, see chapter 20.)

What's a body to do?

There is a move afoot by the National Cancer Institute to get Americans to reduce their fat intake. Their suggestion is to limit fat to 30 percent of daily calories. That's quite a significant drop from the 50 percent typical to the average American, but is it enough? Not according to many who make diet and health their concern. Many suggest limiting fat intake to 10 percent of daily calories.

(For more information on the impact of fats on the body, refer to chapter 4 of *Healthy Habits.*)

TOO MUCH SUGAR

Recent statistics reveal that the average adult American consumes 150 pounds of refined sugars a year. That's 6.6 ounces a day, nearly half a pound. The statistic on teenagers is that they average double that amount. A whopping 80 teaspoons a day! Much of our daily intake of refined sugars comes cloaked in the processed foods we've become accustomed to eating.

For more information on
the impact of sugar on
the body, refer to chap-
ter 9 in *Healthy Habits*.
You will also find a listing of safer sweeteners.
One not listed there is
called stevia. It's much
sweeter than sugar, does
not cause the fluctuation
in blood sugar levels that
sugar does, and contains
no calories. Stevia is a
good choice for diabetics
or hypoglycemics.

"WE"
Na - need 220 - 500 mg
daily

Besides contributing to tooth decay, hypoglycemia, diabetes, osteoporosis, arthritis, yeast infections, and many other disease processes, refined
sugars impair the immune system. Depending on how much sugar has been
recently consumed, the ability of white blood cells to destroy invading bacteria, viruses, and cancer cells can be significantly reduced.

Just 6 teaspoons of sugar, the amount found in about half a can of soda
(the biggest source of teenage sugar consumption), will reduce the killing
power of white blood cells 25 percent over a five-hour period. Twelve teaspoons, equivalent to the amount in a frosted brownie, will drain immune
power 60 percent. A slice of apple pie with a scoop of ice cream, 18 teaspoons of sugar, equals an 85 percent reduction in the killing power of
white blood cells. Finish off a banana split with all the fixin's (24 teaspoons
of sugar), and you'll come close to completely shutting down your protective forces—a 92 percent reduction in your immune system's ability to protect you from the buildup of cancer cells over that five-hour period.[5]

Many of us are walking around with chronically suppressed immune
systems from sugar alone, not to mention all the other immune-suppressing
stressors in our lives. Is it any wonder that soon one out of every two
Americans will experience cancer at some point?

TOO MUCH SALT

The average American consumes sodium to the tune of 4,000 to 12,000
milligrams a day, much of it by way of salt (sodium chloride)—either from
the shaker or from processed foods, where it is found in excess. High
sodium diets are dangerous, especially if you're trying to win back your
health. According to most nutritional authorities, though, the human body
needs somewhere between 220 and 500 milligrams of sodium intake on a
daily basis to function well. This amount can easily be attained from fruits
and vegetables.

The authors of the *Definitive Guide to Cancer* point out that too much
sodium can actually act like a poison to the body—an "enzyme inhibitor."[6]
It's the activity of enzymes that is absolutely fundamental to the well functioning of the human body. Too much salt can bring on constipation—a
forerunner of many forms of degenerative diseases. When salt intake is excessive, fluid in the intestine (which keeps stools soft) is drawn out into the
salty bloodstream. Stools become firm and hard to pass. Waste products
backed up in the colon lead to toxins being reabsorbed back into the
bloodstream, delivering dirty blood to every cell in the body.

Max Gerson, M.D., perhaps one of the best-known pioneers in nutritional therapies against cancer, discovered in his many years of research that cancer patients have a level of sodium in their bodies significantly higher and out of balance with potassium. In a healthy body, these two exist in specific balance with each other.

Because Gerson believed this imbalance to play a key role in the development of cancerous cells, the Gerson Diet (detailed in his book *A Cancer Therapy* and used by thousands around the world to win back their health) includes strict restrictions on salt and other significant sources of sodium, accompanied by potassium supplementation and a vegetarian diet built mainly on fruits and vegetables.

Hypertension (high blood pressure), perhaps the best-known condition attributed to an imbalance between sodium and potassium in the diet, affects an estimated 23 million Americans. Julian Whitaker, M.D., observes: "If your blood pressure reading is above 140 over 90 while you are at rest, you have high blood pressure. Hypertension can lead to blindness, kidney failure, heart attacks, or stroke."[7]

Dr. Whitaker suggests that if you have high blood pressure, think potassium foods: apricots, avocados, bananas, blackstrap molasses, brewer's yeast, brown rice, carrots, dates, dulse, figs, dried fruit, garlic, nuts, potatoes, raisins, winter squash, torula yeast, wheat bran, and yams. And if you have a mind to take some herbal supplements for potassium help, I often recommend alfalfa, horsetail, or hawthorne berries.

(If you need a source, all are available in capsule form from Health*Quarters* Ministries. You'll find our phone number listed in appendix A.) Much more is said about diet and supplements later in this book.

TOO MUCH CAFFEINE

"The Caffeine Anthem"
by Dave Frähm
(sung to the tune of "The Star-Spangled Banner")

Oh say can you see,
my cup of coffee?
It's the stuff that I need
for my fix of caffeine!
Without it I'm a mess,
my head is distressed.
My mind is all shot

CAFFEINE CAUSES
↑ CHOL.
↓ VITS, MINERALS
BREAST LUMPS
BIRTH DEFECTS
OSTEOPOROSIS
KID. STONES
FATIGUE
DIARRHEA
EDGINESS
allergies
Mental problems
destroys B VITS
↓ ability to Fight CA

'til I've had half a pot.
Oh, but now I've found it,
my headache has quit.
My brain has kicked in,
I am human again.
Oh, please don't ever try to take
caffeine away from me.
It's the drug that we crave most,
in the land of the free.

No country consumes more caffeine than the United States. It's in coffee, tea, chocolate, soft drinks, and cocoa. Even some makers of dietary supplements put caffeine in their products. As an herbalist, I recognize that caffeine does have several valuable effects on the body. It can elevate mood, enhance energy, relieve pain, and promote alertness. Later in this book you'll also be learning how to use caffeinated coffee to help stimulate your liver to clean itself out.

Caffeine can be a helpful agent if used judiciously. When I drive my family from Colorado to Iowa for Christmas visits or summertime family reunions, I know that a couple of tall cups of coffee at my side will help me make it through without nodding off.

As long as a person doesn't overuse it, thereby sending his body into addiction, caffeine can be a friend. The problem is that many who use caffeine end up hooked on it. How do you know if you've become addicted? Try going 24 hours without any caffeine (coffee, soft drink, chocolate, etc.). If you get a headache, your body is sending a signal that it's become reliant on caffeine in order to function. You're "hooked."

It's essential to your long-term health to get yourself "unhooked." Regular use of caffeine is a culprit in raising cholesterol levels in our bodies, depleting our systems of vitamins and minerals (particularly B-vitamins and magnesium), and is linked to breast lumps, birth defects (it crosses the placental barrier), osteoporosis, kidney stones, panic disorders, fatigue, and chronic diarrhea.

Without enough magnesium in your body, muscle cramps are likely to occur. Sufficient magnesium stores are also important in order for other minerals to be absorbed into the system.

"Coffee nerves," a condition in which the coffee drinker is on edge, results from the destruction of B-vitamins. These vital nutrients minister primarily to the nervous system and adrenals. Their lack can lead to food allergies, mental problems, and depression. They also play a role in fighting cancer cells and tumors.

(For more information on the impact of caffeine on the body, refer to chapter 12 in *Healthy Habits*.)

TOO MANY CHEMICALS

We now live in a world where most of what we put into our mouths has the potential to bring with it a heavy dose of toxic or otherwise health-challenging chemicals.

Pesticides

Records show that each year in the United States, over 1.2 billion pounds of pesticides and herbicides are sprayed or added to crops. Breaking that down, that's roughly 10 pounds per man, woman, and child.

Are they harmful? You better believe it! Here then are several reasons to avoid pesticide residues by eating only organically grown foods.

Dave's Top Ten Reasons for Eating Organically Grown Foods

1. *Pesticides increase risk of cancer, in general.* The Environmental Protection Agency (EPA) considers 60 percent of all herbicides, 90 percent of all fungicides, and 30 percent of all insecticides carcinogenic (cancer causing). It ranks pesticide residues in the food chain as the third leading cause of cancer within the scope of environmentally derived risks.

2. *Pesticides increase risk of breast cancer.* The rate of breast cancer in the United States has doubled since the 1940s, when the chemical industry started to boom. Organochlorines, one of three main classes of chemical pesticides, are highly fat soluble, and have long half-lives. They accumulate in the breast tissue of women, and they never go away. Studies have shown that they can imitate estrogen's action, tricking the body into producing cancerous cells.

3. *Pesticides increase the risk of prostate and testicular cancer.* Reflective of the increase of breast cancer since "Better Life Through Chemistry" got its start in the 1940s, prostate cancer has doubled, and testicular cancer has tripled. A growing number of studies strengthens the link between these cancers and exposure to agricultural pesticides.

Research done in 1991 showed that "men with prostate cancer have a several times higher level of pesticides in their prostate tissue than men with benign prostatic hypertrophy but no cancer."[8]

4. *Pesticides increase the risk of non-Hodgkin's lymphoma.* "The National Cancer Institute found that the herbicide 2,4-D was associated with a threefold increase in the risk of non-Hodgkin's lymphoma in Nebraska farmers and a sixfold increase in Kansas farmers exposed for more than 20 days per year."[9]

Although this study was done on farmers who were actually working with and handling these toxic chemicals, the importance of keeping pesticides off our dinner plates seems only too obvious.

5. *Pesticides increase the risk of Parkinson's disease.* A team of Canadian researchers found that the major agricultural region of Quebec had almost six times the rate of Parkinson's disease as the areas in the province with the least pesticide use.[10]

6. *Pesticides are linked to inability of couples to conceive.* Dioxin, one of the most potent poisons known and used as a herbicide, is a powerful suppressor of sperm production.[11]

7. *Pesticides increase the risk of birth defects in offspring.* Pick up the latest literature concerning the dangers of pesticide use in modern agriculture, and without exception there will be reference to the fact that pesticides have been implicated in the occurrence of birth defects.

8. *Pesticides have a magnified impact on children.* Because of the size and weight of children, the pesticides found in conventionally grown produce have a greater impact on their bodies than on the bodies of adults. This is particularly problematic for carcinogenic pesticides, since cancer could be initiated more readily during the periods of rapid cell division occurring in infancy and early childhood.[12]

9. *Pesticides increase the risk of psychological and neurological problems.* Exposure to pesticides and herbicides "can give rise to a number of psychological and neurological symptoms including depression, headaches, mental confusion, mental illness, tingling in the extremities, abnormal nerve reflexes and other signs of impaired nervous system function."[13]

10. *Pesticides reduce the nutrient levels in crops.* Researchers at Rutgers University reported that nonorganic (sprayed) produce had as little as 25 percent as much mineral content as organic (nonsprayed) produce. The scientists compared beans, cabbage, lettuce, tomatoes, and spinach purchased at a supermarket and an organic natural foods store, finding substantially higher levels of phosphorus, calcium, magnesium, potassium, sodium, boron, manganese, iron, copper, cobalt, and other minerals and trace elements in the organic produce.

Antibiotics

In today's world of livestock raising, factory farming is the norm. Whereas in yesteryear animals were allowed to graze freely about the farm, today they are often kept confined to pens from birth to slaughter. In such an environment, disease can run rampant. Antibiotics are used regularly to help prevent disease outbreaks from wiping out entire animal populations. Of the 31 million tons of antibiotic drugs produced annually in the United States, half are given to animals.

As a result of this overuse of antibiotics, researchers tell us that antibiotic-resistant strains of bacteria are now showing up in cattle, hogs, and chickens and that these disease-producing strains are transferable across species lines.

Even fish farming, the fastest-growing sector of U.S. agriculture, is experiencing the problems and dangers of overuse of antibiotics. Eric Hallerman, of the Department of Fisheries and Wildlife Sciences at Virginia Polytechnic Institute, says that concentrated conditions in fish farming, just as in factory farming of land animals, often lead to the outbreak of diseases. The use of antibiotics in fish farming is rising rapidly, with the result that drug-resistant bacteria have already been found in fish waste. And just as with land animals, fish diseases can be transmitted to the people who eat them.

Estrogens (Growth Hormones)

The goal in livestock management is bigger animals, quicker. Growth hormones are routinely fed to animals to fatten them up quickly for market. Estrogens are part of that menu. These hormones become concentrated in the animals' fat and tissues and are passed on to humans who consume animal products. Unfortunately, an overabundance of estrogens in the body has been shown to be a significant contributor to many cases of breast cancer.

Food Additives

The book entitled *Safe Food,*[14] prepared by the Center for Science in the Public Interest, lists the "top 10 additives to subtract from your diet." These include:

Other Voices

We are the first generation to eat so many processed foods. Up to 25–75 percent of the nutritional value has been removed from processed foods so that they will have a longer shelf life. This is a vast experiment in what the human body can endure.

SHERRY ROGERS, M.D.

Nitrates (harmless) + bacteria = Nitrates (harmful!)

Nitrates (in Meat) + Heat = Nitrates

1. Acesulfame K
2. Artificial colorings
3. Aspartame (commercially sold as Equal or NutraSweet)
4. BHA
5. BHT
6. Caffeine
7. Monosodium glutamate (MSG)
8. Saccharin
9. Sulfites
10. Nitrites/nitrates

All of these have a track record of being a threat to human health. With some, the threat includes contributing to the onset of cancer. Sodium nitrates have been used for years to preserve meats by inhibiting botulism-causing bacteria. However, bacteria in the meats have a way of turning harmless nitrates into nitrites. When nitrites combine with compounds called amines they form nitrosamines, powerful cancer-causing agents. This chemical reaction can take place both when such meats are subjected to high heat like frying and also in the stomach where nitrites combine with the naturally occurring amines found there.[15]

TOO MANY REFINED FOODS

Food production takes many forms. As fresh whole foods move from harvest to ingredients in various food products, a huge majority of nutrients are lost or purposefully removed—and all for the sake of shelf life.

Suppose you had 26 dollar bills sitting next to you on a table, and while you weren't looking someone came along and snatched them. Later, to show his remorse, the thief quietly slipped four of them back on to the table. Would you be happy about this situation? Would you feel "enriched"?

That's exactly what happens to so-called enriched flours. In the process of creating white flour (done for shelf life and thus monetary purposes), 26 essential nutrients are removed from the grain, along with the bran and sometimes the germ. The law allows manufacturers to put back just 4 of these 26 important nutrients and can then call it "enriched."

Good health comes from the garden and from foods in a form as close to the way God made them as possible. To fill grocery carts with refined and denatured foods on a continuous basis is to commit robbery of our own bodies.

TOO MANY COOKED FOODS

The average American today goes 7 to 14 days without eating any raw fruits or vegetables. The average family of four spends less than two dollars per week on raw produce. Cooked foods, in spite of the fact that they render comfort, are lacking on three important fronts—enzymes, alkalinity, and nutrients.

Lack of Live Enzymes

Every system, every process, every chemical reaction in our bodies is carried on via the action of enzymes. They are to your body what spark plugs are to your car—catalysts that get things started and keep them going. Running and supervising every action in the body, enzymes also help to digest food and work to build, revitalize, and regenerate our cells and systems. In that light they are rightly referred to as youth workers. They assist with internal "house cleaning." They break down toxic substances in our bodies so that we can flush them out without damage to our organs.

There are two broad categories of enzymes in this world: (1) metabolic enzymes found in humans and animals, and (2) plant enzymes. We continually use up our own metabolic enzymes to keep our bodies running. We can make more, but the building materials for this process are live enzymes from an outside source that our bodies convert into metabolic enzymes.

Raw foods have such live enzymes. Cooked foods don't. At 112 degrees, live enzymes begin to die. At 130 degrees, they're gone. If we eat a diet of mostly cooked foods, we fail to supply our bodies with needed supplies for replenishing our enzyme bank account and deplete our enzyme reserves in order to digest what we've eaten. Every time we eat cooked foods we rob our bodies of enzyme power.

Joel Robbins, M.D., uses the example of a young calf to underscore the importance of enzymes to health. Take its mother's milk and heat it to the point of killing all the enzymes, then feed it back to the calf as its only food, and within a couple of months it will die.[16]

The same sort of process happens in the human body when we fail to

Too much protein, fat, sugar, salt, and caffeine and too many chemicals, refined foods, and cooked foods in the standard American diet (S.A.D.) are a grouping of "rocks" that weigh heavily upon the body's ability to maintain health. If you're fighting cancer, change your diet! If you want to avoid cancer, change your diet!

supply it with live enzymes from raw foods. Organs become less and less efficient on a downward slide to a chronic degenerative state.

(*Note:* There are enzyme supplements that can be taken to help supply the body with live enzymes. But supplements are just that—supplemental. It's important not to rely heavily on enzyme supplements in place of making raw foods a lifestyle.)

Lack of Alkalinity

All foods burn down to either an alkaline or acid "ash" in the body as the result of digestion. Included in the category of acid-producing foods are any foods that have been cooked or heat processed. These burn to an acid ash even if they would produce alkaline if eaten raw. For instance, a raw tomato burns to an alkaline ash. Cook it, and you have an acid-producing food.

The standard American diet, built around meat and dairy, is high in cooked foods, thus contributing to acidic conditions in the body. To this add the fact that every cell in our bodies makes its own acid as a normal by-product of energy production. The result is an acidic internal environment.

A body in good health, however, is slightly alkaline. Since our bodies don't make alkaline, it must be supplied from our diet. Raw foods, in particular fruits and vegetables, are our best source.

Lack of Nutrients

Heat destroys nutrients in foods—no doubt about it. The higher the heat and the longer its application, the greater the loss of nutrients. In thoroughly cooked food virtually all the vitamins have been destroyed, along with most of the minerals. The proteins will have been either destroyed or transformed into forms difficult for the human body to digest. Estimates are that cooking destroys about 85 percent of the nutritional value in a food.

Where nutrients are reduced in the diet, so is the power of the body to maintain health.

4

TOXIC DENTISTRY

THE SEVEN WOUNDS OF TOXIC DENTISTRY

THERE ARE AT LEAST FIVE areas of concern that define toxic dentistry as practiced by many in the profession today. The sixth on my list, fluoridation, is a wound administered both in many dental chairs and via many public water systems in this country. The seventh, temporomandibular joint syndrome (TMJ), although often a condition initiated by the body itself, is sometimes the result of poor dentistry. It, too, is discussed here.

- Mercury amalgams (silver fillings)
- Root canals
- Cavitations
- Bio-incompatibility of dental restoration materials
- Electrogalvanism
- Fluoridation
- Temporomandibular joint syndrome (TMJ)

MERCURY AMALGAMS

In dentistry, the word "amalgam" refers to mercury mixed with other dental metals (commonly copper, tin, zinc, and silver) to form a compound for filling decayed teeth. Mercury makes up about 50 percent of an amalgam. If you've got silver fillings in your mouth, you've undoubtedly got mercury in your teeth.

So what's the problem?

1. *The mercury in amalgams is not just toxic, but extremely toxic!* Science has shown mercury to be more poisonous than lead, cadmium, or even arsenic. It is the most toxic nonradioactive inorganic heavy metal known to man. So dangerous is it that it is actually illegal to bury it in the ground. And we let dentists bury it in our teeth?

2. *Amalgams do leak mercury!* Throughout the life of an amalgam, it is continually releasing mercury. Dr. Hal Huggins, a dentist and leading advocate for getting mercury out of dentistry, points out that even apart from chewing, mercury vapor is continuously freed by electrochemical reactions with other metals within the filling. "It then enters the body through the gut, lungs and directly up nerve axons to the brain. . . . It attacks the nervous system, immune system, kidneys and the intestinal functioning because it is an intracellular toxin."[1]

   Huggins states that studies show that certain organisms in the gut convert this released elemental mercury into methyl mercury, which is one hundred times more toxic to the nervous system than the elemental form and passes brain and placental barriers. It's also absorbed 45 times faster and retained longer in the body.

3. *Mercury toxicity can be an underlying cause behind degenerative conditions and diseases.* Mercury released from amalgams binds with certain naturally occurring substances in the body that exist in almost every enzymatic process. Since enzymes are at the core of life, responsible for initiating and overseeing every function of the human body, mercury has the potential of disrupting every system and function in the body. It rapidly depletes the immune system, which protects the body from cancer and other degenerative conditions, and will cause cell damage at the most fundamental level—DNA.

4. *Mercury toxicity is implicated in Alzheimer's disease.* Mercury easily crosses the blood/brain barrier—the brain and nervous system's natural de-

fense against many toxic substances. Mercury toxicity has been implicated in brain-related diseases, including Alzheimer's. Germany and Sweden already acknowledge this reality and have banned mercury from dentistry in those countries.

Alzheimer's disease is considered by most to be incurable. However, a fellow named Tom Warren had success in reversing the disease in his own body and has written a book, *Beating Alzheimer's* (Avery Publishing, 1991). Along with changing his lifestyle and diet and taking specific nutritional supplements, the most important thing Tom did was to seek out dental care to remove the toxic load of mercury he'd been carrying around in his teeth at levels that would shut down industries.

5. *Mercury toxicity can cause mental illness.* You've no doubt heard the phrase "mad hatter" or "mad as a hatter." It comes from yesteryear when makers of fur hats used to hold their creations over mercury fumes in order to waterproof them. Because of continued exposure to mercury, many went "mad" (insane).

6. *Mercury toxicity can cause kidney damage.* In studies in which animals inhaled mercury vapors, the uptake of mercury was greatest in the kidneys (followed by the brain, heart, intestine, and liver, in that order). Mercury has been shown to reduce kidney filtration by 50 percent.

7. *Mercury toxicity can cause multiple sclerosis (MS).* Dr. Hal Huggins, mentioned earlier, a dentist in Colorado Springs and a pathfinder in the movement to get mercury out of dentistry, has over a period of many years consistently witnessed improvement in a majority of MS patients as they've had their amalgams removed. He notes clear symptomatic and laboratory test improvement in 80 to 85 percent and has often seen wheelchair patients who have not been wheelchair-bound for long walk again.

In an article in *Alternative Medicine Digest,* Huggins tells the story of Gonzalo, a 32-year-old highly athletic former soldier who had become wheelchair-bound, almost immobilized by multiple sclerosis.[2]

He had 25 mercury fillings in his mouth. . . . [P]roblems began when he pushed himself a little too hard with his triathlon training. He became paralyzed from the waist down and ended up in the hospital for ten days under examination by three neurologists.

His conventional doctors informed Gonzalo, a former Green Beret, a man believing himself capable of "handling anything," that he was facing a life of chronic, debilitating illness. . . . Instead of languishing into the kind of mental and physical "rot" his doctors insinuated was his future, Gonzalo researched the medical literature. He read about the toxic effects of mercury fillings and remembered that he had gotten sick following the placement of his last three fillings, and that two months after his latest filling and a record-breaking run he'd lost strength and feeling in his legs.

After having Huggins remove all the poisonous mercury fillings from his teeth and replacing them with nontoxic dental materials, Gonzalo not only freed himself from his wheelchair but within three years was back running triathlon races.

For him, the combination of the buildup of mercury toxicity in his body—a concept known as mercury retention toxicity—coupled with physical overexertion had sent his immune system into collapse.

8. *Mercury toxicity can cause heart and circulatory disease.* Soviet researchers have discovered that mercury avidly binds with certain protein sites in the heart muscle that are responsible for its squeezing ability. It could well be that enlarged hearts and heart failures for which there are no known cause are the result of mercury's mischief in the body.

9. *Mercury toxicity can worsen autoimmune diseases such as lupus.* Autoimmune diseases are characterized by a body's immune system being "tricked" into attacking the body's own tissues. In tests on animals, exposure to mercury initiated such auto-antibody production more than 90 percent of the time.

10. *Mercury toxicity can cause birth defects.* Methylmercury, the organic form of mercury that forms in our bodies after we absorb it from our amalgams, is one hundred times more toxic than the elemental mercury actually used in the amalgams themselves. Mercury in this form easily and quickly passes the placental barrier from mother to fetus. Damage caused by this walloping load of toxicity can include mental retardation and stillbirth.

Europe Leads the Way Away from Mercury

In understanding and taking action to protect people from the dangers of mercury amalgams, several European countries are making dramatic strides. Sweden banned the use of all mercury amalgams in children and young adults in June 1995 and extended that ban to adults in January 1997. The

Swedish government, after a study involving 250,000 Swedes, came to the conclusion that immune and other health disorders were clearly related to the existence of mercury amalgams being used in dentistry.

Germany, Denmark, and Austria are not far behind. The German health ministry first recommended in 1991 that the German Dental Association no longer allow amalgams to be placed in children, pregnant women, and people with kidney diseases. They later revised the list of restrictions to include all women of child-bearing age, pregnant or not. At that point the German Dental Association became so worried about potential lawsuits that they said if any additional limitations were forthcoming, they would have to suggest to their member dentists that the use of mercury amalgams be eliminated altogether. Having heard that, a company called Degussa, Germany's largest producer of amalgam and the world's largest producer of metals for dentistry, completely shut down its amalgam production.

What of the United States?

Biological dentistry, concerned with dental treatment and therapies that cause the least disturbance to the immune system, is catching on in the United States. More dentists are reaching the common-sense conclusion that putting toxic metals like mercury into a person's teeth creates a time bomb for an explosion of health problems.

As it does in so many areas of life, though, the din of the "almighty dollar" tends to drown out all other voices. When firmly entrenched behind that din is a political juggernaut like the American Dental Association (ADA), wielding all of its muscle and might in behalf of self-preservation, change comes hard. I say self-preservation, for if the ADA ever came out and openly admitted that putting mercury in people's teeth was a bad idea, I would guess that the number of lawsuits would no doubt radically change the economy of the United States.

Interestingly enough, Dr. Thomas Levy, medical director of Peak Energy Performance in Colorado Springs, points out that in the early 1800s the National Association of Dental Surgeons actually advocated the elimination of mercury amalgam.[3] But its cheapness kept many dentists using it in spite of its toxicity. The Association disbanded several decades later, and the precursor to today's American Dental Association, the National Dental Association, came into being, proclaiming amalgam's safety.

Not surprisingly, the growing number of dentists who are moving toward a "holistic" or biological approach to dentistry—rejecting the conventional view that the mouth and teeth are somehow independent from the rest of the body—are under fire from the ADA. Because of this, some tend to keep a low profile. Those who raise their hands to suggest needed changes, and then go about making those changes in the face of longstanding tradition, tend to get their hands slapped—or even worse.

Hal Huggins, the Colorado dentist, was one of the first modern-day practitioners to incorporate into his thinking and practice what Dr. Weston Price, another dentist, had been discovering and writing about way back in the 1920s—the importance to the entire body of nontoxic dentistry.

Unfortunately, until Huggins came along to force the issue, Price's meticulous research had been largely ignored for 70 years, buried by his critics.

Huggins lists these reasons for getting mercury out of dentistry:[4]

1. It inhibits the repair of DNA, our basic genetic material.

2. It alters the ability of cells to selectively allow materials through their membranes.

3. It changes the three-dimensional shape of molecules, producing nonfunctional chemicals.

4. It alters the activities of enzymes needed to catalyze all biochemical reactions in the body.

5. It interferes with the transmission of nerve impulses from the brain to the rest of the body, and thus produces tremors, shaking, tingling, or numbness.

6. It can provoke the immune system to mount an autoimmune response against its host body.

7. It interferes with endocrine gland function and hormonal secretion.

8. It can displace and deactivate vital minerals such as calcium, magnesium, zinc, and chromium.

9. It kills "friendly bacteria" in the digestive tract, preventing absorption of nutrients.

10. By creating new strains of bacteria, it may make people antibiotic-resistant.

For his efforts, Huggins has been raked through the courts by the ADA and had his clinic shut down. The ADA has also seen to it that in Colorado it is illegal for a dentist to remove mercury amalgams simply for health reasons. The only way it can be legally done is if the client says they're ugly and wants them removed for vanity reasons. When I went to see my dentist, I had to sign a paper that said I was indeed getting my amalgams changed to another substance because I thought them unattractive.

Change is hard. "Change makers" take a lot of heat, especially when change threatens to turn an entire industry on its ear. But before Huggins lost his practice, he'd trained hundreds of dentists who are now practicing biological dentistry throughout the country. An exciting new awareness is beginning to bloom in the world of dentistry. I believe that the next great advancement in modern medicine in the United States will come from dentists and that that advancement is already here.

ROOT CANALS

As dangerous to one's health as are mercury fillings in one's teeth, root canals may be even worse. When decay has burrowed its way through the enamel of a tooth and through the next layer called dentin and finally reached the pulp where the nerve and blood vessels are located, conventional dentistry says, "Time for a root canal."

To make a long, painful story short, root canal therapy involves the hollowing out and filling of an entire tooth. The hope is that by removing the pulp, and thus the nerve, pain will be alleviated and the structure and function of the tooth saved.

Root canal therapy is becoming more and more common worldwide. In the United States alone, dentists are performing the procedure to the tune of 26 million times a year.

What's the Problem?

1. *Bacteria make a home inside the tooth.* Your mouth is always filled with a variety of bacteria. Bacteria play an active role in the tooth decay process. As enamel is eaten away, bacteria enter the more than three miles (if laid end to end) of tubules that form the dentin in a single tooth. When a tooth is hollowed out as part of root canal therapy, disinfectants and antibiotics used to supposedly sterilize the inside of the tooth have no impact on the bacteria holed up in the tubules.

   "They are hardy beasts," writes Dr. George Meinig, D.D.S., in *Root Canal Cover-Up*, "and are polymorphic—that is they mutate, change form. They become smaller in size and number and can then thrive in the absence of oxygen. At the same time, they become more virulent and their toxins much more toxic."[5]

Root canal teeth, then, manufacture and store powerful toxins that if unleashed on your body add to the overall load your immune system has to deal with. The question becomes whether or not these toxins are actually able to leave the tooth.

2. *Exotoxins migrate from the tooth to the rest of the body.* Exotoxins are poisonous chemicals excreted by bacteria. In a July 1997 article in the *Townsend Letter for Doctors and Patients,* Dr. Huggins pointed out that in recent studies more than half of the periodontal ligaments (which hold roots of teeth to bony socket) examined when root canal teeth were extracted contained exotoxins. They had migrated from bacterial infection inside the root canal tooth.

Once these toxic chemicals escape the tooth, they come into contact with the jawbone and its blood supply and can eventually be transported throughout the entire body.

CAVITATIONS

Cavitations are air pockets within the jawbone. They result when a dentist fails to remove the periodontal ligament after tooth extraction. Ligament tissue prevents a complete filling in of bone while a thin layer forms over the top of the socket.

What's the Problem?

Whatever bacteria and toxic substances were in the ligament tissue itself or floating around in the mouth before the pocket was sealed become trapped in the jawbone. Chronic infection and the development of exotoxins result. Antibiotics do little good against these bacteria and the toxic chemicals formed. This constant source of toxins has the potential over a period of time to weigh heavily against the immune system, as the poisons produced seep out into the rest of the body.

BIO-INCOMPATIBILITY TO DENTAL RESTORATION MATERIALS

Bio-incompatibility simply means that the stuff being used to fill cavities in your teeth is causing an allergic reaction in your body.

What's the Problem?

Allergic responses can prove to be severe, putting a heavy burden on your body's ability to maintain health. Reactions noted in various studies have included the development of food allergies, lack of energy and the onset of chronic fatigue syndrome, chronic sinusitis, headaches and migraines, tendency to develop chronic inflammatory changes (including rheumatoid arthritis, phlebitis, and fibromyalgia), development of chronic neurological illnesses, disturbances to the immune system, and a lowering of the pain threshold.[6]

ELECTROGALVANISM

Think "battery." The saliva in your mouth, because of its mineral content, conducts electricity. When it connects dissimilar dental restoration metals in your various teeth (silver-mercury fillings and gold, for instance), a battery effect is created. Even similar-looking fillings placed on different days can involve differing composition and thus create the battery effect.

Since teeth contain fluid, the effect can even be created within a single tooth where dissimilar metals have been placed. A nickel crown placed over an amalgam filling is one such example. Actually, an amalgam, with its blend of dissimilar metals, has the potential to initiate this battery effect all by itself.

What's the Problem?

The electrical charges bouncing back and forth between dissimilar metals in a person's mouth can lead to an electrical impact on your brain and eye tissues.

"Electrogalvanism," says Dr. Edward Arana, "is frequently the cause of lack of concentration and memory, insomnia, psychological problems, tinnitus, vertigo, epilepsy, hearing loss, and eye problems, to name but a few."[7]

Another problem has to do with chemical impact on the entire body. Dr. Arana points out that high dental currents cause erosion of the metals involved, leading to problems of toxic accumulation of metal residues elsewhere in the body. These will destroy tissues and generate disease processes.

FLUORIDATION

Fluoride is the salt form of fluorine, a highly reactive, nonmetallic, toxic element. It was first artificially introduced into public water systems in the United States in 1945. A dentist named H. Trendley Dean had been researching why some people had higher than normal levels of staining on their teeth. He concluded that it had to do with the presence of naturally occurring fluoride in their drinking water. He also concluded that it was this same fluoride that caused these people to have fewer cavities than most—that fluoride makes teeth stronger by actually replacing calcium in their structure, making them harder, more acid-resistant, and less likely to decay.[8]

By the 1950s government sponsorship of the fluoridation of local water supplies was in full swing. Today 62 percent of the country's municipal water systems are artificially fluoridated. Fluoride is also an ingredient in 95 percent of all toothpastes manufactured.[9]

What's the Problem?

1. *Toxic industrial waste is used.* The fluoride being used in public water systems is an industrial by-product from the manufacture of fertilizer and aluminum products. Instead of having to pay $1.40 a gallon to dispose of this toxic waste, manufacturers are able to sell it at 35 cents a gallon to be added to water systems throughout the country.[10]

2. *Fluoridation is rejected by most of the rest of the industrialized world.* If fluoridation is so important to your dental health, why have most of the rest of the industrialized nations deemed it worthless, including Austria, Belgium, Denmark, Egypt, France, Germany, Greece, Holland, India, Italy, Luxembourg, Norway, Spain, Sweden, and Japan?

3. *Fluoride is a poison.* If you saw it in a bottle it would have a skull and crossbones on it, warning of danger. And although the amount ingested in artificially fluoridated drinking water or toothpaste is relatively small, it has been shown to accumulate in the body.

4. *Fluoride inhibits the work of enzymes in the body.* These are responsible for all chemical reactions and are thus referred to as the spark plugs of life. When they can't do their job properly, the whole system goes into steady degenerative decline.

5. *Fluoride can cause ulcers.* When fluoridated water is consumed, it changes the naturally occurring hydrochloric acid in the stomach into hydrofluoric acid, a caustic and destructive substance that can cause serious change to the digestive tract.

6. *Fluoride can lead to hip fractures.* A number of studies show a direct relationship between long-term consumption of fluoridated water and hip fractures in older men and women.

   "Epidemiological studies have repeatedly found a direct relationship between hip fractures in men and women and the percentage of them drinking fluoridated water," writes Julian Whitaker, M.D. "For 30 years fluoride was actually advocated as a treatment for osteporosis, yet we now know that although fluoride promotes new bone formation, it causes the new growth to be weak and of inferior quality."[11]

7. *Fluoride can cause cancer.* Fluoride affects the synthesis and repair of DNA. The result is that fluoride may well contribute to the transformation of normal cells into cancerous cells.[12] Researchers at the University of Texas studying the impact of fluoride on the human body have said that "[t]he terrifying conclusion of the studies was that fluoride greatly induced cancer tumor growth. If doctors and the public can be made aware of this catastrophe, fluoridation shall quickly end. It will some day be recognized as the most lethal and stupid 'Health Program' ever conceived by the mind of man."[13]

   Colorado Springs doesn't put fluoride in the water here. It's already naturally fluoridated. And of the twelve regions that the city is divided into, eight have fluoride levels of one part per million or more. That's already high enough to cause cancer in those who drink it. The authors of *Definitive Guide to Cancer* point out: "Fluoride can produce cancer, transforming normal human cells into cancerous ones, even at concentrations of only 1 PPM (part per million)."[14]

8. *Fluoride can cause neurological impairment.* Two studies done in China showed strong evidence that children who drank fluoridated water had a measurable decrease in IQ compared with those whose water did not contain the chemical.

9. *Fluoride can cause collagen problems.* Fluoride disrupts the synthesis of collagen and leads to its breakdown in bone, tendon, muscle, skin, cartilage, lungs, kidney, and trachea.

Other Voices

10. *Fluoride can cause death from toothpaste overdose.* In 1997 the FDA mandated that fluoridated toothpaste tubes carry this warning: "If you accidentally swallow more than used for brushing, seek professional help or contact a poison control center immediately."

This warning was the result of more than 11,000 calls a year to poison control centers around the country and three fluoride-related deaths. The makers of Crest toothpaste admit to the fact that a family-sized tube contains enough fluoride to kill a child. If your toothpaste is fluoridated, KEEP IT UNDER LOCK AND KEY! Better yet, switch to a brand without the poison.

TEMPOROMANDIBULAR JOINT SYNDROME (TMJ)

TMJ is the misalignment of teeth, jaws, and related muscles, which forces the body to make adaptations in order to efficiently chew food. It is possible for a dentist to actually initiate TMJ in a client by fitting that person with poorly designed dental restorations—fillings, caps, various appliances. It is also possible for TMJ to result from the loss or wearing down of teeth or from abnormalities within the natural growth process as the person matures. It is even possible that electrogalvanic currents caused by dissimilar metals in the mouth are to blame.

What's the Problem?

Adaptation has consequences. When there is misalignment in the bite, the whole cranium will take up the challenge. This loss of symmetry and balance in the mouth and jaw area can lead to a number of unpleasant conditions—headaches, neck pain, lower back pain, even depression and insomnia. It is amazing how one small part of the body, when askew, can make other parts feel the impact.

AND THE GOOD NEWS IS?

Several years ago I made it my unabashed intention to never again grace the reclining chair of a dental office. From my days as a youth, even the thought of something so mundane as a simple checkup sent shivers down my spine. With my family's change to a health-promoting diet, I thought that maybe I could remain dentist-free for the rest of my days. It's a powerful thing that can happen when a little well-placed information begins to eat away at a heavily fortified opinion. If a person is not careful, a new openness can overtake him, making him ready to once again face something he swore he'd never return to.

That's why, a while back, when I could've been doing any number of more pleasant things, I made my first trip in years to see a dentist. I'd been learning the stuff you just read. My dental "challenges" weren't many—just a handful of amalgams—but I wanted them out.

What was my experience like?

I was so eager about taking this major step toward better health that the thought of needles and drills could not deter me. After years of avoiding dentistry like the plague, what I had learned about mercury in my mouth made the opportunity to have it removed an adventure.

Pain? Not like I'd remembered. Somehow, the needles had gotten smaller.

And did I notice any improvements in my health?

I did. I'd been having increasing chronic pain in my left elbow and both shoulders. A doctor friend considered it quite likely that my symptoms were linked to mercury leaking into my system. Sure enough, almost immediately I was symptom free. If you're feeling a bit depressed about how your own dental work may be impacting your health, look on the bright side. At least now you know what might be one of the biggest "rocks" in your "trunk." It's hard to get well if you don't know what's making you sick.

In chapter 13 you'll find information about how to find appropriate dental help.

FURTHER READING

Available from Health*Quarters* Ministries (See Appendix A)

Alternative Medicine: The Definitive Guide, by the Burton Goldberg Group (Tiburon, CA: Future Medicine, 1993), pages 80–96.

Alternative Medicine Definitive Guide to Cancer, by W. John Diamond and W. Lee Cowden with Burton Goldberg (Tiburon, CA: Future Medicine, 1997), pages 980–989.

It's All in Your Head: The Link Between Mercury Amalgams and Illness, by Hal A. Huggins (Garden City Park, NY: Avery, 1993).

Available Elsewhere

Root Canal Cover-Up, by George E. Meinig (Ojai, CA: Bion, 1996).

Toxic Metal Syndrome, by H. Richard Casdorph and Morton Walker (Garden City Park, NY: Avery, 1995).

The Toxic Time Bomb, by Sam Ziff (Santa Fe, NM: Aurora Press, 1984).

5

TOXIC EMOTIONS

MUCH HAS BEEN SAID about the connection between mind and body as concerns human health. The correlation is ancient knowledge. Since biblical times God has made it clear to those who cared to listen that thoughts and emotions can and do impact a person's physical well-being.

"A heart at peace gives life to the body," writes the biblical author, "but envy rots the bones."[1]

Positive emotions can and do help to promote good health. Likewise, negative emotions, if allowed to "fester and ferment," can and do contribute to the onset of illness and disease.

THE BIOCHEMICAL IMPACT OF NEGATIVE EMOTIONS

Research studies have identified that when negative emotions are unresolved and allowed to rule over a person's ongoing response to life, they create potentially harmful disruptions to body chemistry.

Aggressive hostility triggers the release of stress hormones that send the body into red alert—the "fight-or-flight response." That's OK if you're in need of running for your life, but many in today's modern world experience the hormonal rush brought on by anger outside an appropriate context.

Witness the phenomenon known as "road rage"—angry drivers using their cars as weapons to defeat fellow motorists who have supposedly "wronged" them. Anger of this type has the potential to do great internal harm to the body, and cause accidents.

A person continually governed by negative emotions in everyday life is again and again igniting chemical reactions in his or her body that have been shown to have a direct impact on the development of various disease processes.

Redford Williams, M.D., director of behavioral medicine research at Duke University and coauthor of *Anger Kills,* observes: "Getting angry is like taking a small dose of some slow-acting poison every day of your life."

"ORGAN-GRINDERS"

Scientists who study how the mind impacts the body have actually found correlations between the "poisons" generated by specific negative emotions and the particular body organs they tend to impact most.

For instance, if a person carries around unresolved anger, liver function is often negatively impacted. Since this organ is in charge of cleaning blood and sending nutrients throughout the body (besides several hundred other important functions it performs) it's not much of a surprise that unresolved anger has such a devastating impact on one's overall health.

The liver is arguably the most important organ for fighting cancer. I can't tell you the number of times I've talked with participants at our Health*Quarters* Lodge concerning the impact of poorly handled anger. As our discussion progresses, there are always some who identify that "this or that" long-standing anger-producing situation has been a key instigator of their current health problems.

Truly, anger that is allowed to take up permanent residence in a person's mind is a "cancer" in and of itself. It is a huge "rock" that weighs heavily against the healing system of the body.

Next door to the liver lies the gallbladder, a reservoir for bile produced by the liver. It tends to serve as a collecting point for cellular disturbances caused by bitterness and resentment stemming from stored-up anger. The phrase "That really galls me" reflects the connection between resentment and the gallbladder.

As yet another example, no doubt you've heard it said of people that they "died of a broken heart." Unresolved grief truly can, and often does, impact the good working of the heart.

The negative emotions listed on the left tend to affect the organs listed on the right if not dealt with in a health-promoting way:

Anger	Liver
Bitterness, resentment	Gallbladder
Grief, sadness	Heart/lungs
Disgust	Stomach
Vulnerability, feelings of abandonment	Small intestine
Inflexibility, defensiveness	Large intestine
Low self-esteem, feelings of rejection	Spleen/pancreas
Fear, terror	Kidneys
Irritation, timidity	Bladder
Confusion	Thyroid/adrenals

WHAT OF REPRESSED NEGATIVE EMOTIONS?

Repressing an emotion is when you pretend you're not angry and that the wound you've received or the wrong you've felt somehow doesn't matter. You are angry, and it does indeed matter—at least to you. You are allowing your negative emotions to "eat your lunch."

Such behavior makes for mental/emotional problems. Emotions can become so deeply repressed that we no longer mentally remember them, although our cells and tissues continue to be physically impacted by the negative electrical charges and poisons they produce.

W. John Diamond, M.D., coauthor with W. Lee Cowden, M.D., of *Definitive Guide to Cancer,* observes: "Repressed emotions, if not vented or expressed, will seek physical expression, such as functional bowel disease, fibromyalgia, or even cancer."[2]

What's a Body to Do?

In my experience in helping people do what I call emotional cleansing, I've come across two potent mind-detoxifying agents. You'll read more about them in chapter 11—forgiving and thanks-giving. The point here has been to simply highlight the toxic potential of negative emotions on physical health. In other words, to identify the "rock."

6

TOXIC

ENVIRONMENT

THERE ARE HUNDREDS, if not thousands, of things in our environment that can negatively impact one's health. I will focus on the Infamous Five—five environmental challenges to human health common to most Americans. I believe that if you can effectively protect yourself from these five, you'll be doing your body's ability to regain and maintain health a great favor.

- Indoor air pollution
- Water pollution
- Electromagnetic fields
- Excessive sun
- Parasites

INDOOR AIR POLLUTION

Take in a big breath. The single most important nutrient for human life is oxygen, the stuff found in air. Every day we each take in over 17,000 breaths of it. The Earth is currently home to about six thousand billion tons of air. Quantity-wise, we're doing fine. Quality-wise is another story.

In today's world, many of the 17,000 servings we each feast on daily contain contaminants that stress and poison our systems. Dirty air can lead to

- Diseased lungs and a congested liver
- Dirty blood delivered to every cell in the body
- Illness and disease

Since most of us spend 90 percent of our time indoors, whether at home or at the workplace, the air of greatest concern is that found inside the "four walls" of our lives.

A revealing but little known government study tested indoor air quality against outdoor air in seven different communities over a period of several years. They ranged in size from tiny Devils Lake, North Dakota, to sprawling Los Angeles. Participants were given masks to wear that measured pollutants in their indoor air. Results were then compared to samples of outdoor air in their respective communities. Without variance, the pollutants from indoors were always higher than outdoors.[1]

"Many times we are better off outdoors than in the privacy of our own homes," writes James F. Balch, M.D. "Indoor air ranks fifth in the list of top environmental risks to health and, according to the Environmental Protection Agency, it can be up to 100 times more polluted than the air outside."[2]

The average American home contains as many as 70,000 different chemicals that are "outgassing" (being emitted from) the hundreds of thousands of manmade products found there. New carpet can outgas as many as 60 chemicals, some for up to 15 years, while paint can emit 20 chemicals into indoor air for months.[3]

Anytime you breathe in gaseous pollutants they are absorbed into the bloodstream via the lungs. These absorbed pollutants must be filtered out of your bloodstream via your liver. If your liver is also being asked to remove chlorine, fluoride, and other chemicals from the water you're drinking and production chemicals and pesticides from the food you're eating, chances are it will become overwhelmed and sluggish.

I can't tell you the number of times I've talked to someone who came down with cancer within months after moving into a new home. The outgassing from all the manmade products is an incredible "rock" in one's trunk.

As for the "workplace," it's estimated that one-sixth of America's commercial buildings are "sick"—overloaded with airborne toxins that can make their human inhabitants sick.[4] And then there are our schools. Studies

The silver fillings in your mouth are at least 50 percent mercury. If you haven't already read chapter 4, "Toxic Dentistry," about their danger to your health, now would be a good time to do so.

show that one out of every five children attend a school with poor indoor air quality.[5]

The Environmental Protection Agency (EPA) lists three groups of indoor air pollutants that should concern us most:[6]

- Respirable-size particles
- Gaseous pollutants
- Radon

Respirable-size Particles

The EPA describes these as tiny solid or liquid substances that are light enough to float suspended in air. They include larger particles like dust, pollen, molds, and animal dander, plus smaller, invisible particles found in cigarette smoke, unvented combustion from appliances like gas stoves and kerosene heaters, viruses, and bacteria. When these particles penetrate the lungs and respiratory system, they can cause acute or chronic effects, ranging from allergic irritation of the eyes and/or respiratory tissues to more serious effects such as infectious diseases, lung disease, and cancer.

A recent participant at one of our Lodge sessions was a man with Parkinson's disease, a degenerative condition involving the brain and nervous system. Looking back on the various stressors to his health over his lifetime, he identified a primary part of the onset of his illness as undoubtedly his chronic exposure as a research biologist to lead dust in his workplace.

Another participant at the same session, a woman with kidney cancer, had worked for years as a dental hygienist. Looking back at the stressors to her health, she noted that mercury dust had undoubtedly played a big role in the problems she was now facing.

Mercury is one of the most toxic substances on the face of the earth—even more so than lead. In the dentist's office where she'd worked, not a lot had been done to adequately protect workers and patients from inhaling mercury dust floating in the air as teeth were drilled and filled all day long. Once mercury enters the bloodstream via the lungs, it likes to set up camp in the brain, liver, kidneys, and colon. And now here she was with cancer of the kidneys.

Gaseous Pollutants

These include combustion gases and organic chemicals that are not associated with particles. The EPA has been able to detect literally hundreds in indoor air. Sources for combustion gases such as carbon monoxide and nitrogen dioxide include combustion appliances, cigarette smoking, and exhaust fumes from vehicles stored in attached garages.

Gaseous organic compounds find their way into indoor air space via tobacco smoke, building materials and furnishings, paints, adhesives, dyes, solvents, caulks, cleaners, deodorizers, personal hygiene products, waxes, hobby and craft materials, and pesticides. The impact on one's health from these gaseous pollutants can vary from simple irritation of eyes and respiratory system to liver problems, immune and nervous system problems, and cancer.

A past Lodge program participant was an elementary school teacher. Every time she and her students entered her classroom, they noticed strong odors. Many of the kids suffered congestion and runny noses that would clear up almost immediately when they left the room. Best guess? Formaldehyde.

This is the biggest toxic offender in homes and office buildings and can outgas for up to 20 years from the three thousand–plus building and consumer products that now contain it.[7] It's widely used as a bonding agent and preservative in synthetic building products—things like plywood, particle board, paneling, veneered cabinets and furniture, countertops, and so on.

Guess what? The schoolteacher had her classroom in one of those mobile units that so many schools are now putting alongside the main building. And what are they made of? That's right—plywood, particle board, and paneling.

Most of us are swimming in an indoor pool of formaldehyde. It is used in some shampoos, lipsticks, toothpastes, eye makeups, perfumes, hair sprays, nail polishes, soaps, toilet tissues, milk cartons, facial tissues, grocery bags, adhesives, caulking compounds, ceiling tiles, floor coverings, paints, stains and varnishes, car bodies, household disinfectants, curtains, carpets, upholstery fabrics, linens, insulation, and more.

Formaldehyde even puts the "permanent" in permanent press clothing and the "strength" in wet-strength paper towels. It can cause asthma, respiratory allergies, skin diseases, and cancer. Even SIDS (sudden infant death syndrome) has been linked to the outgassing of toxic chemicals, including formaldehyde. What do expectant parents do to the nursery? They get new stuff—new paint, new carpet, new wallpaper, new furniture, new crib, new bedding, new mattress pad, and new clothing. When the baby finally arrives home, her new environment can be a literal gas chamber, too powerful for her immature lungs and liver to handle.

Radon

This is a well-publicized radioactive gas (odorless, tasteless, invisible) that produces particles that may be breathed into the lungs. It originates from the natural breakdown of uranium in the earth's crust and has the potential to cause lung cancer in humans. The risk increases with the level of radon gas in the air and the frequency and duration of exposure.

The EPA estimates that as many as 20,000 cases of lung cancer a year can be attributed to radon poisoning.

WATER POLLUTION

While air is our most important nutrient, water is second. Somewhere in the vicinity of 70 percent of your body weight is water. In an average-sized American adult that's about 12 gallons, requiring consumption of about 10,600 gallons over a lifetime to maintain.[8] It's in your brain, your eyes, your limbs. Every cell in your body contains water.

Just as the air we breathe today can often contain things that challenge human health, so can our drinking water. Studies of both municipal and well water supplies show that what comes from our faucet may contain any or all of the following: lead, mercury, aluminum, cadmium, organic solvents, bacteria, viruses, parasites, industrial chemicals, pesticides, asbestos, radon, nitrates, chlorine, fluoride, and sodium.[9]

Water in America is toxic chemical soup. Apart from all the pollutants we dump into our water supplies, even the chlorine we use to try to clean it up is a major health risk. Studies show that drinking chlorinated water brings with it a 20 to 40 percent increase in the development of colon and rectal cancer.[10] It is also associated with an increase in the risk of bladder, prostate, and other cancers.[11]

Taking showers in chlorinated water can be even more of a threat to health than drinking the stuff! Conservative calculations indicate that inhalation exposures can be significant. Studies show that a person can be exposed to just as much by inhalation during a shower as by drinking two liters of water a day.

Then there's the toxic fluoride some feel we must add to our water supplies, a topic covered in chapter 4.

Are you drinking tap water? STOP! Your liver is charged with filtering poisons from your bloodstream. "Tap water," says Joseph D. Weissman,

M.D., in his book *Choose to Live,* "should be consumed internally only for survival, when good water is not available and you are in danger of dehydration."[13]

Get that? Tap water is bad water!

As Dr. Andrew Weil points out, "It is common for chlorine-resistant viruses and parasites to be able to slip through the more than one thousand large systems in this country lacking proper filters."[14]

In mountainous states like Colorado, where much of our water supply comes from mountain stream runoff, microscopic parasites known as *Giardia Lambia* are common. Awhile back I had the opportunity to view a drop of my own blood using dark field microscopy (see chapter 32). Sure enough, there they were. Parasites. The guests I was harboring were of the microscopic variety, making their way into various red blood cells and hollowing them out. Not a good deal. I made a promise to myself then and there to do regular "parasite purges" (see chapter 17) and to make every effort to stay away from tap water. I also got a water filter for home use that would protect my family.

ELECTROMAGNETIC FIELDS

In today's world, electromagnetic fields (EMFs) are all around us. Wherever there is an electric current, there is a corresponding electromagnetic field being generated. We live in a society populated by electric wires and devices that make our lives easier—but in some cases shorter.

The human body is electrical. You can hold your hand out in front of you and move your fingers. What's happening is that an electrical signal you've generated in your brain is being sent to the fingers to signal movement. The beating of your heart is another example. In this case electrical signals are again being sent but this time apart from your conscious choice.

Scientists have been able to actually measure the electrical current produced within the human brain. The ideal voltage, also referred to as frequency, ranges from 8 to 20 Hz (Hertz, or cycles per second) while awake and can drop to as low as 2 Hz during sleep.

At the same time, the electric "gizmos and gadgets" that surround us— electric stoves, microwave ovens, household appliances, electric blankets, heating pads, computers, copying machines—plus the power lines that deliver electricity to our homes and offices—run on 60 Hz, a much more powerful current. In turn, they radiate a much more powerful electromagnetic field around them than does the human body, although the human body does have one.

In a body consistently exposed for long periods of time to strong electromagnetic fields, cells can be damaged. With all the other threats to the body that the immune system must protect against, it may not be able to catch up to and destroy all the potentially damaged and mutant cells caused by ongoing EMF exposure.

Measuring EMFs

At Health*Quarters* Lodge sessions, I bring two devices into the classroom along with my gauss meter. Gauss is the name given to a unit of magnetic field strength. With my meter I can measure the strength (gauss) of an electromagnetic field being generated by various devices.

The first device I use is a radio alarm clock—the type often used next to beds. If I plug it in and bring my gauss meter within about four feet of it, the reading begins to rise. The closer I get, the higher the reading.

The measurement at which an EMF becomes dangerous to humans is currently in hot debate, but there are many who contend that levels as low as 0.2 milligauss may be harmful. Guess what? At four feet from the radio, my meter already reads 0.2 milligauss.

The obvious conclusion is that if I slept with this radio alarm clock four feet or closer to my head, I would be exposing my brain to potentially destructive EMF stress. Suppose this was ongoing for a number of years. Could it help cause a brain tumor or other brain dysfunction? Many doctors and scientists say yes.

The other device I show people is a paper shredder—the kind that fits over an office wastebasket. Turned off, little if any EMF is radiated. Turned on, it jumps to 3.5 milligauss, but only within a foot or so of the machine. Of course, I'd have to get close to use it, but I'd only be using it for a few brief seconds each day. No big threat, but then there is a transformer on the end of the cord that plugs into the outlet behind my office chair. Even with the shredder turned off, the gauss reading of the EMF emanating two feet from the transformer is 9.2 milligauss. And remember, many claim that 0.2 milligauss is the threshold of dangerous exposure. For several months I'd been exposing my kidneys to potentially significant EMF stress without realizing it.

With anything electrical in your home, field strength coupled with proximity and your length of exposure are key. The electric lamps I own give off next to no EMF. I can sit near them while reading for extended periods of time without worry. But the heating pad I own jumps to 27.7 milligauss when turned on. Needless to say, I no longer use it to coax an aching body into slumber.

Electric blankets present a similar potential threat. The EMF radiating within six inches from them can be as high as 200 milligauss. In some of the newer kinds, that's been reduced to 20 milligauss, still much too high. If you use an electric blanket, warm up the bed with it before you get under the covers, then unplug it before crawling in. Electric blankets, like so many electric devices in our homes, have a "trickle current" running through them even when turned off. Even though this is a much reduced level of current, hours of consistent exposure within close proximity has been shown to have a negative impact on the body.

Another electronic mechanism that most of us have in our homes and offices is a computer. Since many of us spend hours in front of monitors, we need to be aware of the pattern of the EMF they emit. I have noted that the highest readings from my monitor come within the first 12 inches from the screen. At 12 inches they've dropped from a near-screen high of 5.5 milligauss to 2.0. Another six inches back and my reading drops to near zero. If you're concerned about the exposure you're receiving from your own computer, make sure your keyboard is at least 18 inches back from your monitor.

Of course, no discussion of EMFs would be complete without acknowledging the potential danger of living or working near the power distribution lines that bring electricity into our neighborhoods. It was in 1979 that research scientists Nancy Wertheimer and Edward Leeper brought forth the first studies that showed evidence that children living or going to school near such lines were roughly twice as likely to develop cancer as other kids.

Since that first groundbreaking study, others have confirmed the results. Whereas EMFs created by household appliances fall off quickly with distance, EMFs generated by power distribution lines appear to remain strong for hundreds of feet. Study after study show significant association between proximity to these power lines and the development of all types of childhood cancers.

Places that carry supplies for electricians will sometimes carry gauss meters. (See appendix B for the address of a catalog through which you can purchase one.) Prudent avoidance of extended exposure to an electromagnetic field stronger than your own makes sense.

Other Voices

Supposing a young married couple is planning a family. I would not advise them to buy a house under a power line or next to a transformer substation, based on the epidemiological evidence.

W. ROSS ADEY, M.D., neurologist

The skin never forgets sun damage. . . . It's cumulative and additive,[16] writes Dr. Deborah Sarnoff, assistant clinical professor of dermatology at New York University.

EXCESSIVE SUN

Two things are true when it comes to the sun. First, daily exposure to sunlight is important to our health. There is a substance under the skin that turns into vitamin D when exposed to sunlight. This is the best and healthiest way to get your vitamin D, which in turn helps your bones retain calcium.

Sunlight also has a positive impact on hormonal balance in our bodies. The hormones released in the presence of sunlight help to lift our spirits, regulate our sleep patterns, and for women help with PMS.

Sunlight also helps to fight cancer. As Julian Whitaker, M.D., points out, "A healthy dose of sunlight has an inhibitory effect on breast and colon cancer risk."[15] But the second truism about the sun is that too much can be a hindrance to health. "Baking your skin," says Dr. Whitaker, "is just asking for trouble."

Ultraviolet (UV) rays from the sun damage the DNA in human skin. Our bodies produce a chemical called melanin that darkens our skin in protective fashion, but DNA damage is permanent and cumulative.

The fastest-growing cancer in the United States today is skin cancer. About 450,000 folks are diagnosed with it every year. Of these, about 5,500 die of malignant melanoma—a particularly deadly form if not detected early. According to Whitaker, the increase in skin cancer is attributable to two things: (1) the thinning of the ozone layer due to pollution, which in turn allows more UV rays from the sun to reach the earth, and (2) people's lifelong worship of the sun.

With the incidence of skin cancer growing as it is, it's clear to see that excessive sun has become a big "rock" in many "trunks." Later on I'll discuss what the difference is between a healthy dose and a not so healthy one.

PARASITES

Most Americans have parasites in residence in their bodies and don't even know it. Growing up in Iowa, I was well aware that it was standard practice for farmers to "de-worm" their cattle and their kids twice a year. Parasites were then, and still are, a given. In recent medical studies it was estimated that 85 percent of the North American adult population has at least one form of parasite living in their bodies. Some put that estimate as high as 95 percent.[17]

Perhaps you're wondering, "If I've got parasites, how come I can't tell?"

The answer to that is twofold. First, it is the definition and nature of a parasite to keep itself from being detected. The word "parasite" comes from a Greek word meaning "one who eats off the table of another." They sneak in and do their best to stay off the "radar screen."

The second answer to the question is that perhaps you're not aware of the signs and symptoms that signal parasitical infestation. In other words, maybe you are being told by your body but you just don't know its language.

Could parasites be a heavy "rock" in your own body, weighing heavily against your ability to maintain health? The truly nasty thing about having parasites "holed up" in your system is not so much that they're stealing nutrients from you, although that's bad enough, but that as a thank you for your hospitality they're leaving behind toxic waste that can actually be the cause of many disease processes, including cancer.

Types

There are over one thousand different species of parasites that can and do live in human bodies[18] and two basic categories into which they can be divided.

The big ones are worms and are observable by the naked eye (although they may be quite undetectable when ingested). They range in size from tapeworms, which may reach 30–40 feet in length, to hookworms and whipworms that resemble small white threads. In between are critters like inch-long pinworms; flukes, tiny flat worms that look like odd-shaped pancakes; and roundworms, which may reach the size of pencils.

A colonic therapist interviewed for a study gave the following list and descriptions of "big ones" that she's seen come out of people during colon irrigations she's administered.[19] Her comment is revealing: "Everyone has all twelve of these worms in them. Everyone! They are in different layers of the intestines."

Here's how she describes what she's seen:

1. Tapeworms. A fellow colleague keeps a gallon jar in her home. It is full of tapeworms she removed from people, some up to three feet long. (Whitish color, flat, transparent skin.)

2. Whiteworms. These come in all sizes. They are often the color of eggshells and look like spaghetti. They turn black as they grow up.

3. Redworms. These look just like the earthworms you see in the ground. They come out of the colon wrapped in balls. One woman I know recently passed one quart of these worms. They were each six to seven inches long. (Here she's no doubt referring to what are normally called roundworms. They are the most common intestinal parasite in the world, with estimates that one billion people are infected with them.)

4. Inchworms. These are thick, black, and bumpy. They are as thick as a fountain pen and two inches long.

5. Blackworms. These are each 1 to 12 inches long. They come out of the colon wrapped around each other with yellow acid water mixed with them. They live deep in the impacted colon wall.

6. Pinworms. These are little tiny parasites that wiggle when they come out. They are about three-quarters of an inch long. At least one child in five has them. They live in the lower intestine and rectum. (Whereas the roundworm is the most common parasite worldwide, the pinworm is the most common in the United States. Itchy anus can be a sign.)

7. Hookworms. These are curved and are each about six inches long. They come to a point at both ends and are shaped like a fish hook. They are grey. One-quarter of the world's population has hookworms. One expert thinks 50 percent of Americans have them. One man lost an entire quart of hookworms out the rectum. They were alive.

8. "Little Fish." They have a round head and tail. They actually swim when they come out of the colon. In many cases, they will try to swim back up the colon. They come out in schools. They are 1/2 inch long.

9. Whipworms (sometimes called threadworms). These are as thin as thread. They are cream-colored and often come out by the hundreds.

10. "Fuzz Balls." These are round and appear to have fur on them. Many cancer patients have these. They are 1/4 to 3/4 inch in diameter and are yellow. In one 84-year-old man, thousands came out.

11. "Spiders." These are a type of parasite that actually look just like a spider. They often have many legs and are colored brown. Some look like an octopus. They are often one inch long.

12. "Stickpin Worms." These are still another type of parasite and look like stickpins. They are one inch long and have a head like a pea, which is perfectly round. The babies are white and the adults are black.

Little Ones

The "little ones" are microscopic. These are single-celled protozoa that, unlike the worms, reproduce by dividing rather than by laying eggs.

In her book *Guess What Came to Dinner*, nutritionist and author Ann Louise Gittleman lists nearly 20 different kinds of microscopic "critters" that tend to find their way into human bodies. Despite their size, this kind of parasite can be deadly. They reproduce rapidly in the GI tract, then attack organs and tissues. Gittleman refers to them as vampires. Unlike the bigger worms, these guys actually destroy tissues.[20]

Sources

There are many, many things and places from which parasites can be unwittingly gathered. Here are but a few.

- *Drinking water. Giardia lambia,* a microscopic organism, is responsible for most waterborne diseases. It is commonly found in mountain stream runoff but also enters public water supplies via human sewage. It is also found in well water. *Giardia* travels in chlorine-resistant cysts and often slips through the less-than-adequate filters in many rural and urban water systems. As *Giardia* set up housekeeping in the human digestive tract, they tend to prevent proper digestion and assimilation of nutrients.

- *Day care centers.* Careless handling of dirty diapers by childcare workers can lead to parasites of many kinds, including *Giardia,* being transferred from one child to another. Parasites can be transmitted by way of hands, toys, shared drinking glasses, toilet seats, sneezes, and so on.

- *Overseas travel.* Visits to countries where sanitary systems are not as advanced as ours used to be what Americans considered the primary source for picking up parasites. They are still an obvious source, but just one among many for Americans.

- *Pets and farm animals.* Animals play host to any number of uninvited critters that take up residence in their fur and saliva. Fleas have been known to carry tapeworms. And at last count, somewhere around 240 infectious diseases have been identified that can be passed from animals to humans.

- *Underwashed produce.* Animal-derived fertilizers used on fields bring parasites with them. Washing produce before eating is an important practice. In some parts of the world even human waste is used as fertilizer. Roundworms are particularly problematic where food supplies are contaminated by human feces.

There are several important reasons to avoid eating head lettuce, also known as iceberg lettuce. For one, head lettuce tends to be a haven for parasites.

Many folks also enjoy watercress in their salads. If it's not washed properly, liver fluke cysts, which like to attach themselves to the watercress as it grows near streams, will be ingested. Once in the human body, the cysts give way to full-blown liver flukes, which, as their name suggests, make their way to the liver to do their damage.

- *Undercooked meats.* The Centers for Disease Control say that tapeworm infection has doubled in frequency within the past ten years, most likely because of undercooked beef. The beef tapeworm averages 13 to 39 feet long. However, the fish tapeworm (from undercooked fish) is the largest of human tapeworms. They can reach 30 to 40 feet in length and produce more than one million eggs a day! The much smaller liver fluke also comes by way of raw fish. Sushi anyone?

It is the larval migration of the pork tapeworm, however, that represents the most dangerous infection of all the tapeworms.

Pork tapeworm causes great harm to the human host when the immature larvae invade the muscles, heart, eyes, or brain. . . . In the brain, the worms can create a condition known as cysticercosis, which can produce seizures and brain deterioration and often is misdiagnosed as epilepsy.21

Roundworm infections are also abundant in meat-eating cultures. As mentioned earlier, roundworms can reach six to eight inches in length (the size of a pencil). They lay an average of two hundred thousand eggs per day and can actually block the intestines.

- *Going barefoot.* Hookworms are often contracted from walking barefoot on infected soil. As they enter the skin, they create itchy patches, pimples, and/or tiny blisters referred to as dew itch. Parasite infestations can be the cause of many illnesses and disease processes to which they're are not often connected by medical professionals. The symptoms of hookworms are often diagnosed as eczema. Bronchitis may also be hookworm larvae passing through the lungs. Other symptoms can include nausea, dizziness, pneumonitis, anorexia, weight loss, and anemia.

Once in the body, hookworms travel the bloodstream to the throat, where they're swallowed. Their goal is to set up camp in the small intestine.

- *Close contact with others.* Parasite authorities point out that sharing a can of soda, kissing (even on the cheek), intimate sexual contact, being exposed to someone else's sneeze or cough, and just shaking hands can be enough contact to spread parasites from one person to another.

"Pinworms," writes Ellen Reeder, "are the most common round-worm in the United States, and inhabit mostly crowded areas such as schools, day care centers and mental hospitals. They can be as conta-gious as the flu, and usually infect several members of one family."[22]

Since pinworms crawl out of the anus at night to lay their eggs, two people sharing a bed in which one of them is host to pinworms will soon being sharing them as well.

Signs and Symptoms

The presence of parasites in the system can cause a host of symptoms that can be related to other potential causes. For that reason, people with para-sitical infestations may not suspect them as the culprit.

This helps to answer the question "If I've got parasites, how come I can't tell?" Maybe you haven't known what to look for. Many of the larger parasites make their home in the small intestine, thus influencing the diges-tive tract and absorption of nutrients. It could be that digestive problems—constipation, diarrhea, gas and bloating, persistent bad breath, irritable bowel syndrome, and the like—are actually signs of parasites.

Parasites of all kinds can and do travel beyond the intestinal tract. Other health problems that may result from parasitical infestations include joint and muscle aches and pains (fibromyalgia), anemia, convulsions, ab-dominal pains, loss of weight, nausea, dizziness, eye problems, allergies, skin problems, nervousness, depression, hyperactivity, sleep disturbances, teeth grinding, weakness and persistent fatigue, immune dysfunction, un-controllable sugar cravings, diabetic tendencies and blood sugar problems, and much, much more.

Parasites don't make their home in the intestinal tract alone. The mi-croscopic kind, especially, move about the body much like bacteria and viruses, sucking nutrients from the cells of any and all tissues and organs. Even the bigger kind can be found in places other than the small intestine, doing their number on your body—shortness of breath in the lungs, inflammation in the appendix, hepatic injury in the liver, peritonitis in the fallopian tubes, and so on. (For a more detailed summary of parasite-related symptoms, see chapter 17.)

Not only do parasites rob the body of nutrients by stealing them from the digestive tract and other cells of the body, they leave behind toxic waste. A chronic parasitic infection secreting an ongoing level of toxins can become an increasingly heavy burden on the immune system. As it weakens, a host of other infections and disease processes have opportunity to take root.

Every patient with disorders of the immune function, including multiple allergies, patients with unexplained fatigue, or with chronic bowel symptoms, should be evaluated for presence of intestinal parasites.

LEO GALLAND, M.D.

7

TOXIC LIFESTYLE

WE AMERICANS DEVELOP many lifestyle habits that can be characterized as toxic. There are four quite common habits that weigh heavily against our body's ability to fight cancer cells and maintain health.

- Smoking
- Alcohol consumption
- Poor sleep habits
- Lack of exercise

SMOKING

Mona came to one of our Lodge sessions to learn how to clean out her body and renew its healing powers. She had been a smoker for years, ignoring the impact it was having on her body. Like everyone else who smokes, she'd learned to numb herself from facing the common-sense fact that lungs and smoke are not on friendly terms. Now, a pleasant woman in her middle years, she was hooked to an ugly oxygen tank on wheels, coughing up monstrous gobs of mucusy goo and blood, and staring down the barrel of lung cancer.

Smoking is a dumb, dirty, disgusting, health-destroying habit. It's as simple as that. It is, according to Andrew Weil, M.D., "the greatest public health problem in our nation because it is the single most preventable cause of major illness." Dr. Weil also notes that "it is also far and away the most serious form of drug abuse in our society, alongside of which the abuse of illegal drugs pales into insignificance."[1]

- Tobacco use kills three million people worldwide each year.[2]
- Tobacco use is the leading cause of preventable disease and death in the developed countries.
- In the United States, tobacco use kills 419,000 people each year (more than all the deaths from heroin, cocaine, all other illicit drugs, auto crashes, homicides, and suicides combined).[3]
- Over 50,000 medical studies have documented the dangers of tobacco.

Folks, if you smoke, make it your all-encompassing goal to stop. Don't give up 'til you've quit for good. If you willfully choose not to stop, you might just as well throw this book away, because you're not truly serious about being healthy.

Smoking Poisons Your Brain

According to manuals of pharmacology, nicotine, the primary addictive agent in tobacco products, is one of the most fatal and rapid poisons. *Webster's* dictionary defines it as "a very poisonous volatile alkaloid . . . the most active constituent in tobacco, from which it is obtained for use as an insecticide."

That's right, nicotine is used to kill bugs! Guess what it does to the brain! Smoking puts this poison directly into brain tissue more directly than intravenous injection.

Smoking Strangles Your Heart

Smoking is slow death by way of suffocation. Inhaling the smoke of a single cigarette constricts blood vessels and hinders circulation by two-thirds for several hours, reducing the amount of oxygen delivered to organs and tissues. Tobacco smoke also contains more than four thousand toxic gases, including carbon monoxide, which further inhibits the blood's ability to deliver oxygen.

One of the first organs to feel the effects of tobacco smoke is the heart.

In *Dynamic Living,* Drs. Aileen Ludington and Hans Diehl point out: "By age sixty, smokers are ten times more likely to die from heart disease than nonsmokers. Over 160,00 coronary deaths a year are related to smoking, about 30 percent of the total."[4]

Smoking Robs Your Bones
A study published in the February 1994 issue of the *New England Journal of Medicine* revealed that the bone density in women who smoked was 5 to 10 percent less than that of their twin sisters who did not smoke.[5]

Smoking Devastates Your Lungs
The inhalation of tobacco smoke causes the membranes in the air sacs in the lungs (alveoli) to break down. The lungs lose their resilience and elasticity. The air sacs become larger, compensating for decreased efficiency. Carbon dioxide becomes trapped. Pressure builds. Breathing is labored and difficult. Bronchial tubes and windpipe lose their elasticity in the constant struggle for air. The once tiny air sacs begin to resemble large balloons. When they are deflated they no longer return to their original size but resemble wrinkled balloons. This is emphysema.

Smoking Wounds Your Eyes
Daisy Chan, O.D., of the Illinois College of Optometry in Chicago, found that smoking one or more packs of cigarettes a day may as much as double or even triple an individual's risk of developing a condition known as age-related macular degeneration (ARMD). She concluded that it takes 15 to 20 years for an ex-smoker's risk of developing ARMD to decrease to average levels.[6]

Smoking Disrupts Your Digestion
The chemicals in tobacco smoke cause an overproduction of gastric juices and can cause severe indigestion. The same chemicals tend to reduce the efficiency of the valve at the top of the stomach (the cardiac valve), allowing stomach acids to travel back into the esophagus—a painful condition known as acid reflux.

Smoking Paves the Way for the Development of Cancer
The most deadly gas inhaled from burning tobacco is reportedly benzo(a)-pyrene. It's a cancer-causing chemical found in car exhaust and factory

smokestack waste. It causes malignant tumors in lab animals and is identified by the American Cancer Society as a prime cause of lung cancer. By many counts, there are at least 28 other cancer-causing substances released through the burning of tobacco products. They include benzine, N-nitroso compounds, cadmium, arsenic, nickel compounds, and a radioactive element, polonium-210.

Smoking Can Lead to Male Infertility or Birth Defects in Offspring

When a man smokes, the sperm he produces are negatively affected. The great destroyers of sperm health in tobacco smoke are nicotine and cadmium (a toxic metal released in the smoke). Sperm protectors are vitamins C and E, plus Co10. Can an infertile man simply supplement his diet with these nutrients and hope to father children without kicking his "butts"? "During my early urology years," writes Dr. Balch, "my interest turned to male infertility. I discovered that all efforts to effect reproduction would fail if the patient continued to smoke."[7]

Smoking Makes You Dangerous

Medical authorities estimate that secondhand smoke (a mixture of exhaled smoke and what escapes from the burning end of tobacco products) is responsible for as many as 53,000 deaths a year. Tobacco smoke released into indoor air contaminates the breathing space of all present with over four thousand known poisons, many of which are cancer-causing.[8]

Published studies also show that smoking by pregnant women increases the likelihood their offspring will have the kind of respiratory problems observed in babies who later die of sudden infant death syndrome (SIDS).

Dr. Claude Hanet of St. Luc University Hospital in Brussels makes the statement that "the baby of a smoking mother should be considered to be an ex-smoker."[9] Newborns whose mothers smoked during pregnancy have the same nicotine levels as adult smokers and no doubt spend their first days of life going through withdrawal.

ALCOHOL CONSUMPTION

You read a lot of things. You hear a lot of things. The truth about alcohol is that just a little might actually be helpful to one's health but consuming more than just a little is definitely destructive.

The questions remain. What's "just a little"? What does "might" mean?

Most of the studies one might read make it clear that women who drink should consume no more than one alcoholic beverage a day and none whatsoever if pregnant. For men, it's two—the distinction due in general to size difference.

Reading the studies, you find information that would lead you to conclude that a little alcohol goes a long way toward preventing heart attacks and strokes by boosting good HDL cholesterol, preventing oxidation of bad LDL cholesterol that clogs and wounds arteries, and discourages the formation of blood clots.

As a nutritionist and naturopath who wants to help people discipline themselves to do all that it takes to get and stay healthy, I remain unconvinced that alcoholic beverages should remain or become a part of anyone's health battle plan. There are too many variables left unexplained, too many authorities questioning the value of the information gained from these studies, and too much evidence that if you play with fire (or in this case fire water), you could get burned.

Stuart Berger, M.D., author of *How to Be Your Own Nutritionist,* writes: "We know that alcohol can boost your HDL-cholesterol levels . . . but we also know that there is more than one type of HDL-cholesterol, and the kind that is elevated by drinking, unfortunately, does not guard against cardiac problems."[10]

We also know that drinking just one beer can be enough in some folks to cause acute liver inflammation. If the liver is on the skids due to alcohol consumption, even if only for a short time, the many vital functions it performs as the biggest organ in the body will naturally impact the health of the whole system. Is drinking alcohol really worth taking the chance with your health?

What the studies do make clear is that if you don't already consume alcohol, you should not start. Whatever health benefits might be connected to alcohol consumption can easily be achieved by other means and are far outweighed by the real and present dangers associated with alcohol consumption.

Alcohol Is Public Enemy #2

After smoking, overconsumption of alcohol is the second leading cause of death in the United States. It's linked to cardiac arrest; high blood pressure; strokes; cancer of the stomach, throat, breast, and colon; cirrhosis of the liver; and accidents and suicides.

> *Alcohol is the strongest and most toxic of the common psychoactive substances. It is a "hard" drug, harder than heroin, cocaine, LSD, and all the other illegal drugs. Our culture promotes and encourages the use of alcohol and gives the false impression that it is not as dangerous as the disapproved drugs.*[11]
>
> ANDREW WEIL, M.D., *Natural Health, Natural Medicine*

Alcohol Robs Your Body of Nutrients

Alcohol destroys B-vitamins, an extremely important family of nutrients. They are absolutely vital to the well-being of the human body—doing everything from aiding digestion to protecting against cancer.

Alcohol Wounds Your Nervous System

B-vitamins, in particular B1, or thiamin, are the nutrients that minister most to your nervous system. Like caffeine and sugar, alcohol burns them right out of your body. Without your Bs, your nervous system is subject to damage.

Alcohol Can Cause Acute Liver Inflammation

Of all the things you don't want if you're trying to win back your health from cancer, you don't want one more thing to challenge the health of your already overwhelmed liver.

Alcohol Is Linked to the Development of Breast Cancer in Women

The National Institutes of Health has concluded that two alcoholic drinks a day are enough to raise estrogen hormone levels in women, thus putting them at greater risk of developing breast cancer. Diet and disease studies done over the last couple of decades show that women who drink, even moderately, have a 40 to 100 percent greater risk of developing breast cancer than women who abstain altogether.

Alcohol Makes You Extremely Dangerous

University of Minnesota researchers report that babies born to women who drank alcohol during the last six months of pregnancy were ten times more likely to develop leukemia during infancy.

"A pregnant woman, I believe, should avoid drinking any alcohol at all," said Dr. Shu, the lead author of the study.[12] For women who drank any amount of alcohol at any time during the pregnancy, the risk of their baby developing infant leukemia increased 160 to 260 percent.

Fetal alcohol syndrome and birth defects also can be caused by a mother's consumption of alcohol during pregnancy.

What About the French Connection?

It's not unusual these days to read articles about how the French have lower rates of cancer and heart disease, a fact often attributed to their consumption of alcoholic beverages—wine, in particular. The truth is it's not the alcohol that's doing the protecting but the "proanthocyanidins," sometimes referred to as pycnogenols. These are compounds derived from grape seeds and pine bark. French wines, specifically the red types, are loaded with grape seed residues.

Proanthocyanidins are powerful antioxidants that protect the human body from the aging- and disease-initiating effects of free radicals. Studies have shown them to have 50 times the antioxidant power of vitamin E and 20 times that of vitamin C.

Does that mean we should all go out and get some red wine for our health? I wouldn't suggest it. First, the boundary between a little and too much alcohol is narrow. Second, you can get antioxidants elsewhere. Adding grape seed extract and/or pine bark extract to your daily program of supplements is a dynamite idea.

At Health*Quarters* we make available a potent blend of the two, in a base of fellow antioxidants—beta carotene, vitamins C and E, the minerals selenium and zinc, plus several herbs with antioxidant properties. It's a product called New Image Total.

POOR SLEEP HABITS

Sleep. We all need it. When deprived of adequate amounts of quality sleep, our health suffers. "Lack of good quality rest," says Andrew Weil, M.D., "is one of the most common causes of susceptibility to illness."[13] Many of the decisions and lifestyle choices we make negatively impact our sleep. On any given day as many as three-fourths of America's population may be struggling to get good quality "z's."

Common sleep problems are as follows.

Too Late

Scientists tell us that our bodies, for reasons not fully understood, biochemically value the hours of sleep before midnight as twice as important as those following. Because modern civilization now has the option to disperse the darkness with synthetic light, many of us fail to cash in on the health benefits built into those pre-midnight sleep hours. Instead we're up late trying to complete projects or watching late-night TV. As a result, the quality of the sleep we're getting is diminished.

"Oh, but I'm a night owl," many will say. "I can't sleep if I go to bed too early."

Yes, but that's because you've trained your body to function like that.

In the long run you would do well to retrain your system to take advantage of the health benefits afforded by an earlier bedtime. And in case you're a goal-oriented person who likes to stay up late because of all you can get done, imagine the motivational boost you'll get by getting up early and putting in nearly half a day's work before anyone else even gets out of bed!

There's a lot of truth in that old saying, "Early to bed, early to rise, makes you healthy, wealthy and wise."

Too Bright

Science tells us that our bodies are governed each 24-hour period by biological rhythms (referred to as circadian rhythms) directly responsive to light and darkness. There is in every human brain a gland, the pineal gland, which might also be referred to as the third eye. As daylight wanes into darkness, the pineal gland produces a hormone called melatonin—the body's primary active agent in producing sleep.

In addition, scientists have recently discovered that melatonin is also a powerful antioxidant—a quencher of free radical molecules that wound other molecules and are the underlying cause of all degenerative diseases. Dr. Jeffrey Moss, writing in the *Townsend Letter for Doctors and Patients,* notes that "melatonin may be the most powerful quencher yet discovered of the most destructive free radical known—the hydroxyl radical."[14]

It's obvious that the mysterious process we call sleep is a time of healing and restoration for the body. The scientists tell us that up to 70 percent of the body's healing takes place during sleep. Melatonin, produced by the pineal gland, is key to this healing process, as it goes after and helps destroy the millions and billions of dangerous free radicals generated in the system during daylight hours.

The thing about the pineal gland, though, is that it's light sensitive. If there's any light in the bedroom, even as little as that generated by an alarm clock or the light from the moon streaming in through the curtains, melatonin production is hindered. In a domino fashion, too much light in the bedroom leads to less melatonin produced, which leads to both poor sleep and inadequate protection and healing from free radical damage to the body.

Too Full

Eating food too close to bedtime is yet another choice that can negatively impact the quality of the sleep you'll get. A stomach in the midst of the hard work of digestion will keep the mind awake into the wee hours of the night. The circadian rhythms mentioned earlier also regulate optimal times for food intake.

From noon to 8 P.M. might well be labeled Appropriation, for this is the time during the day when the body most wants to be fed. Those studying the issue say we would all do well to eat the biggest meal of our day for lunch, giving our bodies several hours to digest before bedtime.

The hours of 8 P.M. to 4 A.M. can be labeled Assimilation. During this "shutdown" time the body uses the nutrients in foods to build and restore itself.

Finally, the hours from 4 A.M. to noon can be called Elimination. During these hours the key interest of the body is to cleanse and eliminate toxic waste products and food debris from the previous day. Although conventional wisdom says a big breakfast is important, it may hinder the body's ability to do its needed housecleaning in the morning.

I'm an advocate of eating fruit and fruit juices in the morning. Fruit, being mostly water, is easily digested (requiring virtually no digestive energies from the body) and loaded with nutrients. A healthy breakfast of fruits is a great way to start the day, especially for those already compromised with some sort of illness or disease. For those not already compromised, the body can handle the stress of harder-to-digest foods like cereals, breads, and so on.

Too Stimulated

No country on earth consumes as much caffeine per capita as the United States. It courses through our blood from such products as coffee, tea, chocolate, cocoa, and colas. Caffeine hastens the using up of B-vitamins in the system. Bs are vital for the proper functioning of the body's nervous system, which in turn impacts sleep patterns. That cola with dinner or the cup or two of after-dinner coffee may well be the culprit behind the sleep problems many Americans experience.

LACK OF EXERCISE

"The trouble with America," someone once said, "is that we stand to bathe and sit to work."

Fact: Most Americans Are Underactive

Less than 20 percent of adult Americans engage in any sort of regular exercise. Of the underactive majority, roughly 55 percent could be categorized

If you're a day sleeper or fly across time zones or complicate the circadian rhythms that govern your system, recognize that this is a burden to your body. If you're fighting cancer or another serious disease process, let me suggest that you seriously consider a change of jobs. Your job is a lifestyle choice. Don't let that choice continue to weigh heavily against your body's ability to maintain health.

as inadequately active, while the remaining 25 percent are completely underactive (total coach potatoes).

Fact: If You Don't Use It, You'll Lose It

Studies show that beginning at age 25, nonexercisers can lose as much as 2 percent of their aerobic (heart and lung) power each year. By the way, aerobic power is the best overall measurement of one's physical fitness.

At ages 35 and 55, respectively, women and men lose bone mass at a rate of 1 percent a year. Each year 50,000 elderly die from complications following hip fractures, while another 50,000 are immobilized for life. Yet studies show that moderate weight exercise has the potential not only to slow bone loss but actually rebuild it.

Fact: If You Don't Lose It, It May Kill You

It's typical of the average nonexercising American to have traded 7 pounds of muscle for 14 pounds of fat by the time he hits 40 years of age. According to the Metropolitan Life Insurance tables of optimum weight, 62 percent of American women and 72 percent of American men are overweight.

Dean Ornish, M.D., points out that "in a recent study of more than 115,000 American women ages 30–55 who were followed for 8 years, those who were as little as 5 percent overweight were 30 percent more likely to develop heart disease."[15]

Being overweight is also one of the leading causes of adult onset diabetes. And studies show that overweight men greatly increase their odds of developing cancers of the colon, rectum, and prostate, while overweight women are faced with increased risk for cancer of the breasts, cervix, uterus, ovaries, and gallbladder.

8

TOXIC MEDICAL PRACTICES AND PROCEDURES

IN THE WORLD of white coats and stethoscopes, there are a handful of practices and procedures that have the potential to weigh heavily against your health if you add them to the load your body may already be carrying around.

- Drugs and medications
- Breast implants
- Mammography
- Hormone (estrogen) replacement therapy

DRUGS AND MEDICATIONS

The study results were revealed in the April 15, 1998, edition of the *Journal of the American Medical Association*. That same day headlines in *USA Today* and other newspapers around the nation blared the startling news: "Drug Reactions Kill 100,000 Patients a Year."

Ironically, these were not medications that had been prescribed incorrectly, nor were they drugs given inadvertently to the wrong patients. They were medically correct pharmaceuticals prescribed in the light of medically correct diagnoses made by medically correct physicians.

Besides this fact, there are two important reasons why making a habit of medicating every ailment can be a heavy stress on your body's ability to maintain long-term health and healing power.

1. Relying on pharmaceutical drugs is like putting Band-Aids on skin cancer: drugs mask symptoms and divert attention from dealing with underlying causes.

2. Medicinal drugs rob the body of nutrients and thus weaken its self-healing and protective systems.

Drugs as Masking Agents

In today's world of health care, drugs relieve symptoms. Headaches are treated with pain relievers. Colds and influenza are treated with antibiotics. People with heart and circulatory problems are prescribed blood-thinning medications. Folks with cancer are given chemotherapeutic agents.

These conditions are all symptoms of a body out of balance—signs that changes need to be made, often in the realm of diet and lifestyle. There's only one disease—toxicity. Like I've said, everything else is just a symptom. Drugs change the experience of symptoms, thus obscuring the need for change.

"When saddled with a diagnostic label," warns Sherry Rogers, M.D., "look for the environmental and biochemical causes, not a temporizing drug that inevitably has to allow new disease to arise."[1]

Drugs as Nutrient Robbers

Drugs and medications are foreign substances to the body that are toxic to the liver and weaken the immune system. Nutrient stores are used up or destroyed as the body works to purge them from the system. Replenishment is hindered as medications block absorption from foods.

"All drugs are potentially dangerous," observes James Balch, M.D. "The more drugs you take and the longer you take them, the more likely you are to be nutritionally deficient."[2]

BREAST IMPLANTS

A woman recently came to Health*Quarters* Lodge to learn how to put into practice diet and lifestyle changes that would help to improve her health and strengthen her body in a fight against colon cancer.

We talked about the various kinds of stressors that may have been overwhelming her immune system's ability to protect her from developing cancer. She wondered if silicone breast implants could have played a part. She was, in fact, on her third set. The previous two pairs had turned to "stone" and been removed. Now this set had hardened as well.

Why had this happened?

According to Sidney Wolfe, M.D., author of *Women's Health Alert:*

> The human body treats any artificial implant as a foreign object, no matter how soft or smooth. In cases of capsular contracture, a woman's immune system mounts an all-out attack on the object, but because it cannot be ejected, the body forms a collagen layer to wall it off. In some women this wall of scar tissue contracts over time. This shrinking scar capsule eventually compresses the implant, causing pain and deformity.[3]

Why had she repeatedly subjected her body to such abuse?

"My husband wants me to have big breasts." And now here she was with colon cancer.

The Dangers of Breast Implants

A foreign object implanted in the body can lead to immune system exhaustion. When God designed the human body, it was given an immune system to protect it from illness and disease. We need to be careful not to do things that thwart its ability to do so.

Breast implants are one more rock that some women are carrying around, weighing heavily against their immune system's ability to maintain health. When the immune system becomes exhausted, cancer cells thrive.

Many breast implants are made of things toxic to the body. In addition to the fundamental reality that anything foreign implanted in the body will be a continual drain on the immune forces, silicone gel implants in particular add the extra danger of being quite toxic.

Silicone gel implants have been linked to autoimmune diseases. Since they were introduced in 1962, silicone breast implants have been placed in the bodies of an estimated three million American women. Many who have had them in for more than seven to eight years (the average latency for silicone-related diseases to appear) are now seeking out medical help for mysterious symptoms that resemble scleroderma, lupus, rheumatoid arthritis, multiple sclerosis, connective tissue disorders, fibromyalgia, and/or other immune dysfunction disorders.

MAMMOGRAPHY

Anne Frähm, to whom this book is dedicated, found a tiny lump in her breast one day. In the world of allopathic medicine, women are encouraged that if they find a lump they should immediately seek out the feedback of a mammogram. She did.

"Noncancerous," was the reply of the physician who read it. "But just in case, let's do an ultrasound." Again his response was "noncancerous—nothing to worry about." Within a handful of months breast cancer had spread to her spine, sternum, ribs, and pelvic bones. Stage 4. Terminal.

Is mammography worth the heavy emphasis placed on it by the conventional medical community?

1. *Mammography is an unreliable source of information.* "Mammograms have been shown to have anywhere from a 20–30 percent false negative, and a 20–30 percent false positive rate," says W. Lee Cowden, M.D., coauthor of *Definitive Guide to Cancer.* "That means they're wrong anywhere from 40–60 percent of the time. Not very reliable."[4]

    A false negative means the test said there was nothing to worry about when in reality there was. A false positive means you had the hell scared out of you, perhaps even went through the emotional agony and expense of a follow-up surgical procedure, only to find that you'd been handed an inaccurate reading in the first place.

2. *Mammography has the potential to actually stimulate the development of breast cancer.* On June 2, 1991, the London *Times* published an article entitled "Breast Scans Boost Risk of Cancer Death." It summarized the results of the Canadian National Breast Screening Study (NBSS), the largest study of its kind ever undertaken.

    For eight years (1980–1988) the study had tracked 89,835 Canadian women who were between the ages of 40 to 49. Half were given mammograms every 12 to 18 months. The other half were simply given a single physical exam. Nothing else.

    At the end of the eight-year period, breast cancer deaths among those who had received the mammograms were 52 percent higher than those who hadn't.[5] Some will argue that radiation used to irradiate breasts at that time was much higher than what is generally being used today. But is there really any safe level of radiation?

No, says John W. Gofman, M.D., Ph.D., a well-known authority on the impact on health of ionizing radiation (the kind that comes from mammography, X-rays, and other medical diagnostic sources). "Our estimate is that about three-fourths of the current annual incidence of breast cancer in the U.S. is being caused by earlier ionizing radiation, primarily from medical sources."[6]

3. *Mammography may well spread existing cancer.* When a woman exposes herself to mammography, great pressure is used to squeeze her breast tissue between two flat plastic surfaces.

   "If there are cancer cells," says Lorraine Day, M.D., herself a breast cancer survivor, "they are more likely to spread to other parts of the body, so that now you have cancer cells circulating in the bloodstream."[7]

4. *Mammography is not actually "early" detection.* It is my opinion that the heavy emphasis put on mammography has led many women to place unfounded confidence in its helpfulness. Not only is it unreliable and potentially dangerous, as I've already pointed out, but it's also ineffective as an "early" warning signal.

   "It takes approximately eight years of growth before a breast cancer can be found on a mammogram," writes Charles B. Simone, M.D., author of *Breast Health.* "During those eight years, many things happen, including the dissemination of those cancer cells to other organs by way of the bloodstream."[8]

5. *There is a potentially more effective, obviously much less dangerous detection tool.* No test is perfect, but some may be better. Instead of mammography (for all the reasons just listed), I would personally opt for the Anti-malignin Antibody in Serum (AMAS) blood test (see chapter 31). This test does not tell the individual where in the body the cancer is located. It simply signals whether or not there is a cancerous process happening. This may at first sound disconcerting. Wouldn't you want to know where the cancer is?

Cancer is a systemic disease. Something has so weakened the system (too many rocks) that cancer cells (which are always with us) have been allowed to thrive. As Dr. Simone has pointed out, once a tumor is actually detectable, cancer cells have already spread throughout the whole body anyhow.

Bottom line: When the goal is to strengthen the body so that the body can heal the disease, it doesn't matter where in the body the cancer is.

HORMONE (ESTROGEN) REPLACEMENT THERAPY

The conventional wisdom in the health field until recently has been to give women who are either perimenopausal (close to menopause), or actually in menopause, hormone replacement therapy using estrogen. The thinking behind such therapy was that the menopausal drop in estrogens was the culprit behind the crippling progressive bone loss known as osteoporosis and was responsible for an increased risk of cardiovascular disease (the leading killer of women).

However, medical science has now discovered two important things:

1. The hormone that needs replacing is not estrogen after all but progesterone. And not just for women nearing or in menopause but for all women 35 years old and over and for all men past their mid-forties. (For more, see chapter 20.)

2. Giving women replacement estrogen is potentially dangerous and damaging.

There are at least three reasons why any woman considering estrogen replacement should do some thorough homework before taking that route.

1. *Estrogen replacement stimulates the development of breast cancer.* Harvard Medical School researchers have concluded that estrogen replacement therapy for postmenopausal women increases their risk of breast cancer.

   "Estrogen feeds cancer while progesterone inhibits it," observes Joseph M. Mercola, D.O. "It would be wise to phase off the estrogen as soon as possible and replace it with natural progesterone. If hot flashes are a problem, a phytoestrogen like black cohosh is generally very effective."[9]

2. *Estrogen replacement does not rectify osteoporosis.* Studies show that while estrogen given menopausal women may help to slow bone loss, it does nothing to help rebuild new bone. "Progesterone and not estrogen is the missing factor . . . in reversing osteoporosis," says John Lee, M.D., the leading "guru" in the United States today on hormone replacement therapy.[10]

   It's important to note here that the synthetic progesterones (referred to as progestins) don't work—or at least not nearly as well. According to Dr. Lee, they are synthesized from natural progesterone for economic reasons by pharmaceutical companies. Natural progesterone, although itself synthesized in a lab environment from plant sources, is an exact replica of human progesterone.

3. *The majority of estrogens being prescribed come from horse urine.* Premarin, the best known and most often prescribed estrogen replacement agent, is derived from the urine of pregnant mares. Horse estrogens work well for horses, not for humans. In the female body they can lead to breast tenderness, headaches, leg cramps, gallstones, worsened uterine fibroids, endometriosis, fluid retention, blood sugar problems, and increased risk of cancer.[11]

TOOLS FOR UNLOADING

Only a detoxified body has both power of resistance and healing.

MAX GERSON, M.D.

NOW YOU HAVE a better idea of the "rocks" we pick up making our way through life in today's world. The amazing thing is not that one out of every two Americans will develop cancer at some point in their lives, but that the other one out of every two of us won't!

Let's talk now about tools you can use to help clean out ("detoxify") your system. This is where the fun begins. Every one of the things in the next ten chapters (with the exception of chapter 13) is something that you can do for yourself to help renew and stimulate your body's God-given healing powers.

- In chapter 9 you're going to learn how to get more oxygen into your system by practicing deep breathing. Oxygen is your most important nutrient. Most of us use only a fraction of our lung capacity for taking it in. Cancer can't survive in a well-oxygenated environment.

- Second in importance is water. It may be that the root of most degenerative diseases is dehydration—inadequate intake of water. The average American is chronically and persistently dehydrated. In chapter 10 I'm going to teach you Frähm's Principles for Water Consumption.

- As you have already seen in chapter 5, there really is a mind-body connection that impacts physical health. In chapter 11 I'm going to present two key tools for cleansing your mind of toxic emotions—forgiveness and thanksgiving.

- Because the liver is of vital importance when it comes to fighting cancer, I'm also going to teach you in chapter 12 how to do a liver/gallbladder flush.

- A dry skin brush is one of the most important tools for you to learn to use on a regular basis. Its health-promoting benefits can be enormous. You learn about these in chapter 14.

- Since your skin is the biggest organ for detoxification, I'm also going to instruct you in chapter 15 in ways and means of soaks and saunas.

- Another key tool in the battle to clean and empower the body is the minitrampoline, also referred to as a rebounder. Many consider this the most important form of exercise for moving lymph fluid through the system. Chapter 16 explains its use.

- It has been estimated that 95 percent of Americans are at any one time infected with parasites. The problem is not in having them, but in not doing anything about them. Left to do their thing, they wound tissues, create carcinogenic waste, and can cause cancer. In chapter 17 I'm going to teach you how to purge them from your body.

- At the core of any program to detox and renew the body is the juice fast, along with colon and liver cleansing. This is the "big gun," the heavy artillery in the war on sickness and disease. At the end of chapter 18 you'll find several charts that will help you put together a daily schedule that incorporates these various "unloading" tools.

9

DEEP BREATHING

AIR, A BLEND primarily of oxygen and nitrogen, is essential for human life. It is the fundamental nutrient. We are more dependent on its oxygen content for our survival than any other element. The human body can go weeks without food and days without water, but just a few minutes without oxygen and we're goners.

As important as oxygen is to our bodies, scientists tell us that most of us utilize only the top 10 percent of our lungs when we breathe. The bulk of our lung structure lies dormant, underactive. If our lungs are not exercised and fully expanded on a regular basis, they will begin to lose their elasticity. The power to expand the chest will gradually diminish.

Failing to give our lungs a proper workout regularly we not only deprive our bodies of increased levels of its most important nutrient, but also grow increasingly unable to fully exhale all of the carbon dioxide and related toxic wastes that the lungs are responsible for removing.

The regular practice of deep breathing is the answer. The average person has a lung capacity of 250 cubic centimeters. With discipline, this can be doubled within a few weeks. Maximizing lung capacity by way of deep breathing exercises increases oxygen levels, which does the following things to minister to the body:

- Alkalinizes the blood and tissues—an important component of good health
- Fights degenerative disease; cancer cells cannot survive in a well-oxygenated environment
- Improves mental powers and alertness; oxygen nourishes brain cells
- Improves circulation
- Relieves stress and promotes a relaxation response

HOW-TO'S

- When deep breathing, always inhale through the nostrils. The nose is a filtering agent, purifying the air we breathe before it reaches our delicate inner organs.
- Imagine that inside you is a balloon. It fills from the bottom up as you breathe in through your navel (use your imagination) and empties from the top down as you breathe out through your mouth. Putting one hand on your chest and the other on your abdomen, the one on your abdomen should be moving more than the one on your chest.

Steps

1. INHALE: Breathe in through your nose, filling your lower lungs first (abdomen and stomach should be expanding), then your rib cage, and finally your upper chest area. Count while doing this.
2. HOLD: Hold your lungs full for as long as you can. Again, count.
3. EXHALE: Slowly exhale through your mouth for the same count as you inhaled, keeping your lips partially closed to produce resistance. Feel the balloon collapsing down, with your stomach the last part to retract.
4. HOLD: Hold your lungs empty for same count as you held them full.

Practice

- Start with one-minute sessions, three times a day. Add one minute to each daily session each new week until each of your three daily sessions is five minutes long. (If all goes as planned, that should be week 5.)
- Work at extending counts for inhale-hold-exhale-hold. For example, if you start with 5-5-5-5, perhaps your next goal might be 10-7-10-7, and so on.

Note: In chapter 22, "Air and Water Purification Strategies," you'll learn how to make sure the air you're breathing deep is clean.

FURTHER READING

Back to Eden, by Jethro Kloss (Loma Linda, CA: Back to Eden Books, 1939), pages 546–551.

Beating Cancer with Nutrition, by Patrick Quillin (Tulsa, OK: Nutrition Times Press, 1994), pages 102, 108.

The Natural Laws of Healthful Living, by Carlson Wade (West Nyack, NY: Parker, 1970), pages 199–211.

Oxygen Therapies, by Ed McCabe (Morrisville, NY: Energy Publications, 1988), pages 202–205.

10

WATER DRINKING

IN THE WAR ON CANCER and other degenerative diseases, keeping your body adequately hydrated is second only to deep breathing. Each of the trillions of cells in our systems is a producer of waste material, the natural by-product of energy production. Without needed fluid, the cells can't flush themselves. As toxins build up, cells begin to break down. Mutations, sickness, and cancer cells result.

HYDRATION FORMULA

To figure out how much water you should drink on a daily basis, here's a simple formula. First, take your body weight and divide by 2. Then equate that with ounces. For a 200-pound man, the body weight divided by 2 gives 100. That's how many ounces he should consume on a daily basis to maintain hydration of the tissues. If the same man wanted to figure out how many 8-ounce glasses that would be, he'd simply divide 100 by 8, giving 12 to 13 glasses a day.

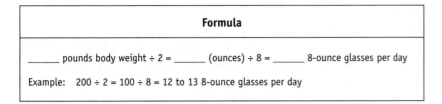

Formula
_____ pounds body weight ÷ 2 = _____ (ounces) ÷ 8 = _____ 8-ounce glasses per day
Example: 200 ÷ 2 = 100 ÷ 8 = 12 to 13 8-ounce glasses per day

FRÄHM'S PRINCIPLES OF WATER CONSUMPTION

1. *Either you buy a water filter or you are one. And in this day and age, you don't want to be one!*

In his book *8 Weeks to Optimum Health,* Andrew Weil, M.D., observes:

> Water is one of the major sources of environmental toxins that can harm your healing system. According to recent reports, drinking water in the U.S. is increasingly becoming a health risk, whether you live in a big city or a rural area. More than 100 million Americans drink water that contains significant levels of three cancer-causing chemicals: arsenic, radon, and chlorine by-products.[1]

Water in America is toxic chemical soup. Even the chlorine we use to try to clean it up is a major health risk. Then there's the toxic fluoride some feel we must toss in, or go around toothless. And in case you thought "critters" in aqua were only a problem in Mexico and other third world countries, Dr. Weil states: "In addition to chemical contamination, chlorine-resistant viruses and parasites can slip through the more than one thousand large systems in this country lacking proper filters."

As I said earlier, if you're drinking tap water in the good old U. S. of A., stop! Your liver, charged with filtering poisons and pests from your bloodstream, is under heavy attack. Add to that all the nasty stuff that enters the bloodstream via air and food, and you've got a liver that may well throw up the white flag.

A liver too overwhelmed to function properly sends dirty blood throughout the body. The garbage our cells were trying to flush out comes back to settle in. Dirty blood means dirty cells means disease. Don't drink tap water! Tap water is bad water!

Bottled water?

You bet. And because bottled purified water is readily available from any number of companies in most cities, you don't need to buy a personal

I'm a big fan of an under-the-counter RO system. I've had one in my home for a number of years and have found it to meet all our needs.

water purification system for your house if you don't wish to. Check your yellow pages.

However, it's wise to stay away from the gallon jugs of bottled purified water in grocery stores. Water is a solvent and tends to leach chemicals from soft plastic containers. The longer it sits in the soft plastic jugs, the more plastic particles will be ingested when you partake. Purchase water stored in heavy plastic or glass containers. Some grocery stores and health food stores have water purification machines on site. Go ahead and fill a few soft plastic jugs if that's all you have, but drink the water within a few days.

Notice I've been using the word "purified"? Stay away from any bottled waters that have not gone through some sort of actual purification process. Check the label. There are bottled waters with pristine-sounding names that come from "mountain streams" or faraway "underground springs," but the purity is questionable. Drink tap water from mountain runoff here in Colorado, and you're quite likely to wind up with an infestation of the microscopic parasites called *Giardia*. Chlorine doesn't kill 'em. The truth is the most reliable water, as far as purity, comes right out of the tap in your home. Put it through a purification process, and you've got good drink.

There are basically three types of water purification processes that have significant value as to their ability to create the purest water: reverse osmosis, distilled, and ozonated. For more information, particularly concerning reverse osmosis (RO) and distilled, refer to chapter 3, "Drink Pure Water," in *Healthy Habits*. An ozonator (not covered in *Healthy Habits*), designed to add extra oxygen to water, is also worth a look as your method of water purification. The additional oxygen has been shown to neutralize chemicals and kill any "critters" in the water. At Health*Quarters* Ministries I've seen to it that we actually carry RO systems for those who wish to purchase one from a trusted source—and at an excellent price. Since we do volume sales, we're able to keep prices low. Call us if you'd like more information; for our number, see appendix A.

2. *TYWBE—take your water bottle everywhere!*
Scientists tell us that as we age we tend to lose our thirst sensation. It is a well-documented reality that most Americans are chronically dehydrated. Not only do we not drink enough water, we guzzle gallons of fluids that, although they do contain some water, contain other chemicals that actually rob the body of what little water we do consume.

Coffee is a diuretic. It draws water from the system. It has been said that for every cup of coffee drunk, the body requires two cups of water to rectify the robbery.

Water is so important to the "unloading" process of detoxing the system that one of the first things we tell our guests at Health*Quarters* Lodge is that if they're not in the bathroom most of the time while they're with us, we're not doing our job for them. That's a bit of an overstatement, of course, but they get the point.

At the outset we hand each guest a bottle filled with purified "liquid life" and point them to the dispenser where they can refill. When we tell them to take their water bottle everywhere, we mean everywhere! We expect to see water bottles lining the floor 'neath the pew on Sunday when we head down the mountain to church. We assure them that God will be pleased to see good stewardship of health going on in His house.

3. *Limit your water intake during meals.*

It's best not to drink too much water, or other fluids, with your meals. You will need to take a little in order to wash down the supplements you'll no doubt want to be taking with meals, and I do believe that supplements are a must. But the problem with drinking a lot of water during meals is that it dilutes digestive fluids produced in the stomach.

Lemon water is known as a natural form of hydrochloric acid—the acid the stomach makes in order to digest fats and proteins. Adding lemon to your mealtime glass of water, then, is an excellent digestive aid.

11

MENTAL DETOXING

Practicing Forgiveness

and Thanksgiving

I KNOW A GIRL who was gang raped. I have a friend who was abandoned as a child. There are people in my life who've been lied to, stolen from, and abused. I know people who have been victims of affairs, women who are mistreated by their husbands, kids who have been beat up at school, and people whose reputations have been cruelly maligned. I don't know anyone who hasn't been sinned against in some way. I don't know anyone who doesn't have something to forgive.

These are the words of Sonia Huenergardt, a nutritionist and friend of Health*Quarters* Ministries, from an article entitled "Forgiveness." She's right. There's not a single one of us who doesn't have something or someone to forgive. You can't go through life without scars.

But what happens if you go through life without forgiving?

In chapter 5 I talked about how negative emotions, if not dealt with in a healthy manner, can cause decay of our physical health. Unresolved or repressed anger is an especially nasty health threat. The internal energy generated by it tends to negatively impact the liver, which in turn impacts the purity of our blood and thus the health of the whole body.

For you and me to be physically healthy in this world, we need to know how to effectively forgive the wrongs that have already been done to us and those wounds that have yet to come our way. As I was searching for words with which to shape this chapter, Sonia's article came across my desk. She captures the essence of what forgiveness is—and what it isn't. With her permission, I share here more of her thoughts.

Having grown up in a Christian home, I am not unfamiliar with the concept of forgiveness. Or the necessity of it. I have tried to forgive people. Sometimes it felt like it was working. Sometimes it didn't. But, quite honestly, I don't think I really understood what I was supposed to be striving for. What is forgiveness, anyway? And how do I know when it has happened?

Forgiving sounds so good and right and holy. But for some reason, it hasn't seemed to satisfy the part of me that demands justice. Something hasn't quite seemed fair about forgiveness. It has felt equivalent to saying, "What you did was OK. There was nothing wrong with it. In fact, you can keep doing it to me, and I'll let you and won't say a word."

I've learned that's not what the Lord means when he asks us to forgive those who trespass against us. When I recently read the book *When We Pray for Others,* I began to understand forgiveness a little bit more.

Forgiveness is canceling a debt. I never understood why the Lord's Prayer in Matthew says ". . . as we forgive our debtors" (King James Version). I could understand transgressions and sins, but debts? Then I realized when someone wrongs me, my offended soul demands restitution. I feel they owe me something. They at least owe me an admission of wrong. Or saying they're sorry. Or suffering a few consequences. Or changing. Or restoring the damage done. Or making it up to me in some way.

When I forgive, I am not saying that what someone did to me was OK. The idea of canceling a debt acknowledges that there was a debt incurred. I have been robbed of something that a Godly relationship would have given me. I am not ignoring that I have been hurt and may need to heal from some scars. I am not saying they were not wrong. It does not mean that I can't take any steps to deal with repetitive problems. It does not always replace the need to talk or resolve the problem. If a crime has been committed, forgiveness does not cancel the civil debt. I simply cancel the person's emotional debt to me. When I forgive, the person's sin against God or government is not canceled. But his or her debt to me is canceled.

I cannot cancel someone's sin. That is God's domain and God's alone. "Never [think] that you own revenge . . . but leave room for the wrath of

God, for it is written, 'Vengeance is Mine, I will repay,' says the Lord" (Romans 12:19, New American Standard Bible). "But You, O God, do see the hurt, the grief and the pain, and You will call that person into judgement and avenge the helpless and the victims" (Psalm 10:14, Today's English Version).

When I forgive, I leave the other person's debt entirely with God—God who is just and the Judge of all the earth. He will take care of all that in the end. I am not waiting and expecting that other person to do something to make it up to me. If they want to do the right thing, they will apologize and do what they can to make it right. Our relationship may never be what it could have been, if they do not. But I may grow bitter waiting for them to "get it together," if I feel they have to make a move before I am willing to forgive.

Releasing someone of their debt to me, whether I verbalize it to them or not, also releases me. It does not deny a problem or the need to deal with a problem. In some cases, I may still need to distance myself from the person or the situation in order to heal. But when I decide to cancel a debt, it frees me to relate to my offender and to deal with the issue without anger, bitterness, grudges, or revenge. It keeps me from falling into criticism and judgment of the person. It allows me to rejoice when God works in that person's life, even when He blesses him or her, without resentment that he or she didn't first pay the debt to me.

Forgiveness is not necessarily easy. Sometimes I have to forgive again and again, as the temptation comes to remind the person of what they did. At times my mind may want to rehearse the offense and my reaction to it, just to reinforce my resentment. Deep hurt summons strong emotions, and I may need to weep with God and struggle through those emotions with Him.

I have heard it said that if I still remember the incident, I have not really forgiven. I don't believe that's true. Through forgiving and healing, however, I can come to the point where feelings of pain and anger do not accompany the memory.

I don't think true forgiveness is possible without the grace of Jesus Christ working in a person's heart. He has promised to be "abundantly available for help!"[1] Love, mercy, and forgiveness cannot dwell in me without Him. When I acknowledge my weakness and cry out to Him, He has pledged Himself to strengthen me.[2]

Jeff Harkins, who wrote *Grace Plus Nothing,* prays along the following lines to help him in the forgiveness process:

In Jesus' name, because He forgives me, I choose to forgive so-and-so [plug in name of individual or group]. I hereby cancel their debt.

Henceforth, they owe me nothing; they never have to apologize; they never have to admit they were wrong. They never have to admit that I was right. I let them off the hook. I cancel their debt. They owe me nothing.[3]

Bottom line, when I forgive I am set free. The restitution my offended soul demands is annulled. My job as bill collector is over. I don't have to labor to right the situation. I will cancel a debt. God will see to it that justice is served. But I will show mercy. After all, I, too, am a debtor.

Holding a grudge. Reinforcing resentment. Demanding revenge. Just a few of the many ways to pour gasoline on the flames of anger. In order to protect yourself from anger's destructive force to your health, particularly your liver, let me suggest that you practice detoxifying your mind by finishing each day with this simple question: "Whose debt do I need to cancel?"

PRACTICING AN ATTITUDE OF GRATITUDE

We had a woman come to our Lodge several years back who had nothing good to say about anything or anyone. Hers was not a pleasant world. Hard as we tried, we couldn't please her. She'd come to us because she wanted to learn how to use nutrition to help strengthen her body against a cancerous process that she had growing in her breast. It soon became clear that her biggest obstacle to good health was a cancerous process that she had growing in her heart—a bitter and complaining spirit.

There truly is a mind-body link. Thoughts do turn into chemistry in the body. Bitterness and complaint, if allowed to fester and ferment, are extremely toxic to the system—a cancer in and of themselves. The poisons they generate weaken a person's ability to regain and maintain physical health.

On the other hand, people who have established in their lives the twin foundations of emotional/spiritual health—forgiveness and now thankfulness—seem to live above it all. These people are like a man I read about who, when he began to practice forgiveness with his parents, found them opening up to him in ways he'd never known. When he added thanksgiving to his daily agenda, his disease process began to fade away, till at last he was free.

Not for all, but for some, it's the deep-seated, undying angers and complaints in life that keep them bound as captives to a disease process.

DEVELOPING A HABIT OF THANKFULNESS

I suggested that you make it a habit to end each day with one simple question: *Whose debt do I need to cancel?*

Help that habit take root in your life with daily doses of thankfulness. Changing your focus from what you lack or have lost to counting your blessings not only helps melt away negative emotions but also is life giving.

Each morning for 30 consecutive days write down five things for which you're thankful. These must be five new things each day. By the end of this exercise you will have made a list of 150 things, and a new habit. Get a notebook and keep going.

12

LIVER/ GALLBLADDER FLUSHING

WANT TO LIVE a long and healthy life? Take care of your liver. Because it carries on its daily chores without fanfare we tend to ignore its importance. When it begins to falter, however, the whole body feels the effect.

The second biggest organ of your body (skin is first), your liver is charged with accomplishing over five hundred vital functions to keep you "in the pink." It converts food into stored energy, supplying the system with the power it needs to maintain life. It is also the key player in the digestion of fats by way of the production of bile (which it stores in the gallbladder for later use).

Your liver also cleans your blood of stuff that would otherwise cause you great physical harm. That stuff includes drug residues; excess estrogens; leftover histamines from allergic reactions; toxins released by bacterial infections; alcohol; pesticide residues; chlorine and fluoride from drinking water; thousands of poisons released in tobacco smoke; and a million other toxins found in the air, water, and food.

When the liver is not working right, the whole body suffers.

What makes for a sick liver?

- *Insufficient hydrochloric acid production in stomach.* Sugar and caffeine deplete the body's stores of Bs. The stomach requires B-vitamins in order to produce hydrochloric acid to enable proper food digestion. When food is improperly digested, toxic gases enter the bloodstream and are delivered to the liver—a cause of major liver stress.

- *Insufficient friendly bacteria in the intestinal tract.* There are "good guy" and "bad guy" bacteria in the intestinal tract. The "good guys" are destroyed by antibiotics, birth control pills, sugar. . . . Without these friendly bacteria, protein residues in the colon putrefy, forming toxic substances that are absorbed through the intestinal wall and delivered back to the liver.

- *Too little fiber in the diet.* Fiber is essential for sweeping the intestinal tract clean of toxic waste. The average American is carrying 7 to 60 pounds of encrusted fecal matter and mucus in his or her "gut." Trapped toxins are reabsorbed through the intestinal wall into the bloodstream and delivered back to the liver.

- *Too much alcohol consumption* depletes the liver of nutrients necessary to carry on its various detoxification functions and "releases dangerous free radical oxidants. The result can be damaging to both the structure and function of [the liver]," according to Jeffrey Bland, Ph.D.

- *Too much acetaminophen (Tylenol).*

- *Too much sugar.* The average American consumes 150 pounds of refined sugars every year. That's 1/3 pound every day—40 teaspoons. It finds its way into our bodies by way of refined food products on our supermarket shelves, most especially by way of sodas.

- *Too much caffeine.* No country in the world consumes as many caffeinated products per capita as does the United States. It's found in our coffee, tea, soda, chocolate, cocoa, diet pills, and so on. Unfortunately, kids are taught to consume caffeine in our school systems, as schools these days are signing contracts with either Coke or Pepsi to carry their brew in school vending machines. We get 'em started early weakening their livers.

- *Too much animal fat (red meats, dairy products, fried foods).*

- *Too many refined foods.*

- *Too many acid ash–producing foods.* All foods burn down to either acid or alkaline ash after digestion. The body needs to remain slightly alkaline to stay in good health. Meat, dairy, and sodas—typical American fare—burn to acid ash.

- *Too many food additives (artificial flavors, colors, preservatives).*

- *Too few veggies.*

- *Too few raw foods.* "When not eating enough raw foods as 50 to 80 percent of the total intake each day, the liver may be developing some clogging," says Corinne Allen, Ph.D., editor of *Charis Nutrition News.*

- *Mercury released from dental fillings.* If you've got silver fillings, you've got in your mouth the most toxic nonradioactive element on earth. It has been scientifically shown to continuously leak over the lifetime of a filling, as much as 80 percent of these mercury fumes being absorbed through the lungs into the bloodstream. Once inside the body, it has an affinity for the brain, liver, and kidneys. Mercury is "cytotoxic," meaning it kills cells. (See chapter 4.)

- *Yeast overgrowth (Candida).*

- *Fungal infections.*

- *Parasites.*

- *Viruses (hepatitis, etc.).*

- *Bacteria.*

- *Immunizations.*

- *Radiation (microwave ovens, computer screens, TV sets, cell phones, etc.).*

- *Emotional stress.*

- *Repressed anger.*

- *Tobacco smoke.*

What are the signs of a sick liver?
(Put a check by those you're currently experiencing.)

- Poor digestion (gas, bloating, acid indigestion, nausea, pain, sense of fullness, cramping)

- Poor elimination (constipation, diarrhea)

- Blood sugar disturbances (diabetes, hypoglycemia)

- Intolerance to fatty food, cooking oils, and spicy foods

- Congestion

- Dry tongue and mouth
- Thick ridges on fingernails
- Jaundiced (yellowish) skin and eyes
- Eye inflammation
- Erratic eye movements
- Red eyes
- Skin boils
- Susceptibility to infection of either viral or bacterial origin
- Headaches
- Dark circles or bags under eyes
- Achy back or pain between the shoulder blades
- Body odor
- Muscle pain (fibromyalgia)
- Liver spots
- General depression and "the blues"
- Unexplained weight gain or tendency to gain weight easily
- Intolerance to sugar
- Intolerance to alcohol
- Elevated bilirubin and/or liver enzymes
- High cholesterol and/or tricglycerides (or too low—below 140 mg/dl)
- Foul-smelling gas
- Extreme fatigue
- Skin itching
- Food allergies
- Sensitivities to chemicals (perfumes, soaps, cleaning fluids, exhaust fumes)
- Sudden hair loss
- Dizziness, shakes
- Female reproductive complaints (scanty menstrual flow, PMS)
- Light-colored stools
- Pale, greasy stools that float
- Cancer (and various other degenerative conditions)

HELP FOR A HURTING ORGAN

Today one out of every two Americans develops cancer at some point during his or her lifetime. However, the truly amazing thing about the health scene in the United States is not that so many are getting cancer, but rather that so many aren't. With the typical American diet and lifestyle stacked against our livers, it's a wonder we don't all die in our thirties and forties.

Luckily, or might I say by God's foresight and planning, a person's liver can take a great deal of abuse before it says, "I quit." It's estimated that the human body can continue to function in reasonable fashion on just 20 percent of total liver capacity—in other words, 80 percent dysfunctional. It's also estimated that by the time the average American eating the standard American diet turns 38, he or she is already functioning on only 35 percent liver function—in other words, 65 percent dysfunctional.

Even so, a person with 35 percent liver function still feels and performs a whole lot better than those who are getting by on just 20 percent. Imagine how great a person would feel at 75 percent function or even 100 percent! It can happen. The human liver can and will regenerate itself to full function if given a chance. That depends on you. It takes dedication to the cause and a great deal of work.

Besides the obvious diet and lifestyle changes that need to be made, coffee enemas (see chapter 18) should be part of "liver reclamation" projects. There are also certain foods and supplements that minister greatly to liver function (see chapters 18 and 19). Another tool to help restore proper liver function is the Liver/Gallbladder Flush—a purging of gallstones.

"One of the leading contributors to impaired liver function is diminished bile flow or cholestasis," write Michael Murray and Joseph Pizzorno. "Cholestasis can be caused by a great number of factors, including obstruction of the bile ducts and impairment of bile flow within the liver. The most common cause of obstruction of the bile ducts is the presence of gallstones."[1] Murray and Pizzorno say the prevalence of gallstones is related to the high-fat/low-fiber diet consumed by the majority of Americans.

It is also true that gallstones tend to form as the result of eating a diet high in acid ash–producing foods. If most of what you eat is acid ash producing, your body will take sodium from the bile stored in the gallbladder to help alkalinize the bloodstream. What it leaves behind is cholesterol, which solidifies into stones. Once the sodium is all gone, the next step is taking calcium from bones. This is where osteoporosis begins—a diet high in acid ash–producing foods.

Regardless of how the stones got there, keeping them is a great threat to your long-term health.

THE HEALTH*QUARTERS* MINISTRIES LIVER/GALLBLADDER FLUSH

You will need:

- Juicer (I recommend the Champion juicer, which is available from Health*Quarters*)
- A good supply of organic apples (Granny Smith are best for juicing)
- 2 oz. cold-pressed, extra virgin olive oil
- 4 oz. lemon or grapefruit juice
- 12-ounce bottle of magnesium citrate (available at drug stores or in the health section of your supermarket)

In lieu of a juicer you will need freshly made organic juices.

Directions

1. For three days drink at least four glasses of freshly made apple juice. The malic acid in apple juice helps to begin to soften and break up stones. It is not necessary to be fasting. However, when you are fasting is the best time to do this sort of flush.

2. On the evening of day 3, drink 2 oz. olive oil mixed with 4 oz. lemon or grapefruit juice.

3. Lie down on your right side for 20 minutes, keeping your right knee as close to your chest as you can. (This position opens the pathway to your gallbladder, so that the olive oil and lemon juice can work to dissolve and clean out any stones that have been forming. A bit of "flu-like" nausea is not unusual but will quickly pass.)

4. Before going to bed, drink a 12-oz. bottle of magnesium citrate.

5. When you awake the next morning (or that night) and use the bathroom, expect to pass what might be referred to as sludge. You might also pass soft, round stones of varying sizes and colors, mostly green. They float, and they look much like fuzzy, undigested peas. Some people have passed hundreds at a time.

13

DENTAL DETOXING

This is a must for
anyone who has
amalgam
(silver/mercury)
dental fillings or
root canals.

BRUCE FIFE, N.D.,
The Detox Book

I DID A NUTRITIONAL ASSESSMENT for a client who had been diagnosed as suffering from a form of epilepsy. He wanted to know what sorts of foods and supplements might help him with energy levels. For about a year he'd been experiencing occasional "seizure-like" experiences—not complete blackouts; more like mild "brain fog" and lightheadedness. Constant ringing in the ears had also become a problem (a condition often referred to as tinnitus). Also on his list of symptoms were chronic fatigue and a frequent need to get up at night to urinate.

As I listened to him tell me what he was experiencing, it occurred to me that each of his symptoms could be signals of heavy metal toxicity in his body. When I asked about mercury fillings and root canals, he showed me a mouthful. Suggesting certain nutrients and herbs with which he might minister to specific organs that were showing nutritional weaknesses, I also suggested that he consider seeing a "biologically trained" dentist to ask about detoxing his dental work.

Biological dentistry stresses the use of nontoxic restoration materials for dental work and focuses on the often unrecognized or overlooked impact that dental toxins and hidden dental infections can have on one's overall health. At the end of this chapter is a listing of organizations to call or write that may be able to link you with such a dentist in your area of the country.

In my ministry of helping folks take better care of their bodies, I've become amazed at how often I see dental work playing a key role in a person's ill health. Hopefully by now you've read chapter 4, "Toxic Dentistry." If not, stop here and go back and read it.

SIGNS AND SIGNALS

The Toxic Element Research Foundation lists the following symptoms associated with heavy-metal toxicity.[1] Any number of these might be experienced by a person carrying around mercury or other heavy metals in the teeth. You'll note that all of the symptoms my client was experiencing are included in this list.

- Unexplained irritability
- Constant or frequent periods of depression
- Numbness and tingling in extremities
- Frequent urination during the night
- Unexplained chronic fatigue
- Cold hands and feet, even in moderate and warm weather
- Bloated feeling most of the time
- Difficulty remembering or use of memory
- Sudden, unexplained, or unsolicited anger
- Constipation on a regular basis
- Difficulty in making even simple decisions
- Tremors or shakes of hands, feet, head, and so on
- Twitching of face and other muscles
- Frequent leg cramps
- Constant or frequent ringing or noise in ears
- Getting out of breath easily
- Frequent or recurring heartburn
- Excessive itching
- Unexplained rashes, skin irritation

- Constant or frequent metallic taste in mouth

- Feeling jumpy, jittery, nervous

- Death wish or suicidal intent

- Frequent insomnia

- Unexplained chest pains

- Constant or frequent pain in joints

- Tachycardia

- Unexplained fluid retention

- Burning sensation on the tongue

- Getting headaches just after eating

- Frequent diarrhea

In addition to all these troublesome symptoms, parasites and yeasts (a parasitical plant)—are drawn to mercury. Parasites will find their way to where mercury has lodged in various organs, bringing with them bacteria, fungi, and viruses. It could well be that the epilepsy-like symptoms my client was experiencing were being caused by a combination of mercury and parasites in the brain tissues.

QUESTIONS TO ASK

Perhaps by now you, too, have recognized the need to make dental detoxing an important part of your own cancer battle plan. Your next step is to locate a biological dentist.

There are four key questions to ask of any prospective dentist to make sure he or she is the kind you're looking for. Many dentists will remove your mercury fillings and replace them with something else yet have no training in the proper procedures. There are precise and important guidelines and safety measures that must be followed—both for your sake and for the sake of the dental staff themselves.

1. *By what means do you determine the sequence in which to replace a person's fillings?* "Mercury fillings act as miniature electrical batteries," writes Hal Huggins, D.D.S.

   Some register a positive charge, others a negative. . . . If you remove the fillings from the mouth quadrant (upper and lower jaws, right and left sides) with the highest negative charge first, then the body will respond optimally; if you take out those with the highest positive charge, the body chemistry will decline rapidly and the symptoms (various ailments) will worsen.[2]

To find out in which quadrant the highest negative charges lie, a properly trained dentist will use an ampmeter, a device capable of registering the highest peak of electrical current emission in the mouth.

Huggins suggests that if you're suffering from leukemia or ALS (amyotrophic lateral sclerosis), even more rigid rules of amalgam removal need to be followed. "You must remove the two fillings with the highest negative readings, regardless of where they appear in the mouth; then you remeasure and remove the next two. You keep going this way until all the mercury filling shave has been taken out."

2. *How do you protect yourself and your patients from breathing in mercury fumes and debris during the process of removal?* Thomas Levy, M.D., medical director of Peak Energy Performance in Colorado Springs, suggests that, at the minimum, protocol standards should include:[3]

- Use of a rubber "dam" (to prevent swallowing of amalgam)

- Operatory room air filtration that can remove airborne mercury from the drilling

Additional precautions include:

- Masks for the staff

- Fresh air tube placed over the nose of the patient

- High volumes of cold water used to minimize exposure to mercury vapor and particles

3. *How do you determine what sort of restoration material to use in place of the removed amalgam?* "Tooth-colored composite fillings are a safe alternative to amalgams," writes Jane Heimlich, associate editor of Dr. Julian Whitaker's *Health and Healing* newsletter. "They're more expensive than mercury-silver amalgams and take longer to place, but they are free of mercury."[4] They are usually made from ceramic material.

Whitaker goes on to point out that while amalgams (which are a blend of mercury with other metals) are the most toxic of all dental materials, all metals used to fill teeth or rectify dental problems have the potential to be harmful. "Fifty percent of American women are allergic to nickel (commonly used in crowns and bridges), and in some people, a combination of metals acts like a 'mouth battery,' creating electric currents that can cause a variety of problems."

A biologically trained dentist, aware that your dental materials must be not only nontoxic but also non-allergy-producing in your body, will pretest all materials for allergy responses before installing them in your mouth.

Heimlich lists the following tests as helpful.

- *Clifford material reactivity testing.* This is a blood test that will tell your dentist which of the hundreds of potential restoration materials would be best suited for your personal chemistry. For more details, you or your dentist can call (719) 550-0008.

- *Electrodermal screening (EDS).* You can read more about EDS in chapter 39. It is the use of a machine that measures the electrical responses of the body when presented with different substances. A person skilled in the use of such a machine can identify which dental materials stress your autonomic nervous system and which ones don't. To locate a dentist or other professional trained in this procedure, contact BIOMERIDIAN, Inc., at (801) 495–1188.

- *Muscle response testing (MRT)* involves the measurement of the same electrical responses of the body when presented with various substances. When clients ask for a nutritional assessment, I use MRT to help identify nutritional stresses and deficiencies, plus dental stresses. (Read more about this in chapter 29.)

4. *What sort of detox protocol do you recommend following amalgam removal?* The type of dentist you'll want to trust your health to will suggest a detox plan for you to follow after your amalgam removal that will help to purge your body of remaining mercury stores.

Typical elements of such a plan include:

- *Chlorella and garlic.* Oral supplements of each help to bind with mercury and flush it from the system. Dietrich Klinghardt, M.D., Ph.D., who is regarded as the chief "guru" on dental detoxing these days, suggests that both supplements be taken at highest comfortable tolerance levels.[5]

    Individual tolerance of chlorella can range from as much as 14 capsules a day to as little as half a capsule. You'll know you've exceeded your tolerance level if you experience nausea, heartburn, diarrhea, and/or headache.

Klinghardt suggests that for the first eight days after amalgam removal, chlorella should be taken with meals (maximum daily tolerance level divided by meals eaten). Then on days 9 and 10 take ten times the usual dose, but not more than 60 capsules in a single day. Days 11 and 12 are meant for rest from chlorella. The next day starts the 12-day cycle over again. Ask your dentist how many 12-day cycles you should do.

As for garlic supplements, Klinghardt suggests that the tolerance level be based on smell. When you begin to be able to smell it on your breath, you've reached your daily limit.

- *Cilantro (pesto or tincture).* Known as coriander or Chinese parsley, cilantro is one of the only substances that will bind with and flush mercury from the brain and central nervous system. There are two ways to increase your intake of cilantro. Klinghardt suggests making a pesto. Put organic cilantro in a blender with water, sea salt, and olive oil. Blend until creamy. Take 1 to 3 tablespoons three times a day with meals. The other way is to purchase a tincture (extract) of cilantro. An excellent source is Dragon River Herbals, at (800) 813-2118.

  Dr. Richard Keller, D.D.S., of the Plantation Center for Craniomandibular Disorders in Plantation, Florida, instructs that after taking a dose, you should rub your middle finger with your thumb for five minutes. This bit of acupressure helps to open up the blood-brain barrier, allowing the cilantro to get into the brain to bind with and flush the mercury found there.

- *Vitamin C and magnesium* help to stimulate bowel movements, which helps to keep mercury moving out of the body in the feces. If the bowel is sluggish, mercury and other toxins have an opportunity to be reabsorbed through the intestinal wall back into the bloodstream.

  Vitamin C should not be taken in oral form in the hours leading up to your dental appointment, since it will neutralize anesthetics used to numb nerve endings. On the other hand, intravenous vitamin C can be used before, during, and after amalgam removal, since it doesn't have the same neutralizing effect.

- *Colon cleansing: enemas and colonics.* Both of these forms of colon cleansing help to ensure the flushing of mercury via the feces.

- *High-potency multi-vitamin/mineral supplementation.* The body will not detox mercury if it is mineral deficient.

- *Chelation therapy.* To "chelate" means to *combine* or *bond with.* Chelation therapy (see chapter 28) is the introduction into the bloodstream of various organic chelating substances (EDTA, DMPS, DMSA) that bind with heavy metals in the body and flush them out through the kidneys.

- *Herbal or homeopathic liver and kidney drainage remedies.*

- *Dry sauna.* Your skin is your biggest organ of detoxification. Exposing yourself to the high temperatures in a dry sauna will help the body push mercury out through your pores. Shower immediately afterward to keep the toxins from being reabsorbed.

- *High-protein diet.* Klinghardt says that "a high protein diet is essential to mercury detoxification."

HOW TO AVOID THE CHAIR

Once you've cleaned out the dental toxins and associated problems in your mouth, let me encourage you to make the necessary changes to keep yourself dentist free. Here are three habits that will help you stay clear of "the chair."

1. Cut way down on sugar and other sweeteners.
2. Move toward more raw fruits and veggies in your diet.
3. Augment your diet with key supplements.

Since it's a well-known reality that today's farming practices have depleted our soils, I'm an advocate of adding dietary supplements to one's daily health routine. The following is a dynamite trio to help to protect and enhance not only your dental health but the health of your body as a whole.

- *CoQ10.* Not only shown to help protect against periodontal (gum) disease but also helps to revitalize the immune system, protect and strengthen the heart and circulatory system, normalize high blood pressure, energize body cells, and increase stamina/endurance.

- *New Image Total.* A potent blend of antioxidants that help strengthen the immune system against bacteria that attack teeth. It also helps the whole body by protecting against toxins, free radicals, inflammation processes, oxidation of cholesterol deposits, and the damage that could be caused by heavy metals in the system (lead, mercury, aluminum, etc.). Contains: pine bark extract, grape seed extract (each 50 times more potent than vitamin E and 20 times more potent than vitamin C) plus quercetin, vitamin C, Siberian ginseng, zinc picolinate, vitamin B6, ginkgo biloba, L-cysteine, silymarin (milk thistle extract), selenium, vitamin E, and beta carotene.

- *Super Supplemental (without iron).* I suggest that a "multi" is the foundation for any program of supplementation. I also suggest that it not contain iron. Not only do bacteria feed on iron, but iron supplementation is usually unnecessary if you're eating a diet of more than just junk foods. Too much iron in the body can lead to excessive free radical formation.

Many of the supplements listed in this chapter can be found at your local health food store. They can also be ordered through Health*Quarters* Ministries.

Resources for Finding a Biological Dentist

Foundation for Toxic Free Dentistry
P.O. Box 608010
Orlando, FL 32860-8010
Website: www.bioprobe.com
For a referral to the closest mercury-free dentist they have on their list, simply send your request to them with an SASE (self-addressed stamped envelope).

Environmental Dental Association
P.O. Box 2184
Rancho Santa Fe, CA 92067
(800) 388-8124 or (619) 586-7626
To receive a list of alternative dentists in your area, send $3 plus a business-size SASE.

Peak Energy Performance
Colorado Springs, CO
(800) 331-2303 or (719) 548-1600
Call for referrals.

Just because a dentist does not use mercury does not mean that he or she knows how to properly remove the mercury already in your teeth. The organizations listed here can help you locate mercury-free dentists in your area, but remember to ask the four key questions I've listed. If you're uncomfortable with the answers you get, keep looking.

Or if you simply want to go somewhere where you know things are going to be done right, check out the Center for Progressive Medicine in Puerto Vallarta, Mexico. Dr. Huggins trains and consults with their personnel on a part-time basis. For more information, call 1-888-843-5832 (Website: www.progressive-med.com).

DRY BRUSHING

DRY BRUSHING IS total body brushing using a dry brush on dry skin. Use of a natural fiber bristle brush is important, since nylon bristles can tear the skin.

WHAT ARE THE BENEFITS?

There are many. In fact, natural health practitioners consider dry brushing an important habit to be practiced on a daily basis.

It helps to clean and detoxify the skin.
Your skin is your biggest organ of detoxification. Healthy skin eliminates up to a pound of toxic wastes every day in sweat. For that reason, it has been called the third kidney. Since skin also breathes, it also has been referred to as the third lung. Dry brushing helps to keep skin healthy, resilient, and free of dead skin cells that contain toxin. When the skin is doing its job, it takes some of the burden off the body's other organs of detoxification—the kidneys, liver, lungs, and colon.

It helps to stimulate and invigorate the body's electrical system.
Thousands of years ago the Chinese discovered that the human body is not

only chemical (blood and saliva) and structural (bones and muscles) but also electrical. Your heart beats due to an internal electrical system. You can move your fingers with a simple thought because of that same electrical system—electrical signals sent from the brain to command movement. Acupuncture and accupressure are two sciences that are based on the electrical system of the body, as are electrocardiogram (EKG) machines that measure heart electricity, electroencephalogram (EEG) machines that measure brain electricity, and lie detector machines (cross my heart!).

There are three million nerve points spread over the surface of your skin, some seven hundred of which are nodal, or "electrical relay stations." Dry brushing of the entire body helps to stimulate these relay stations to keep the current flowing along the electrical lines the Chinese dubbed meridians. In this way, every part of the body is energized and empowered to do its best work.

It helps to move lymph fluid.
Lymph fluid is derived from blood plasma but is clearer and more watery. As blood circulates through the body, lymph fluid seeps through capillary walls to fill the space between cells. All the soft tissue in the body is bathed in lymph fluid. The body has twice as much lymph fluid as blood. Besides this lymph fluid, the lymph system includes lymphatic capillaries and larger vessels—lymph nodes (also referred to as lymph glands), the spleen, the tonsils, and the thymus.

The lymph system does several important jobs for the body. Filtering out disease-causing organisms, producing white blood cells and antibodies, and distributing fluid and nutrients throughout the body, it also removes excess fluids, proteins, and debris that are squeezed out of capillaries as blood circulates through the body. The lymph system is part of the disposal system of the body. Lymphatic capillaries collect debris-filled lymph fluid and return it to the bloodstream at two points near the top of the chest. In this way wastes are removed by the liver or kidneys and excreted.

Unlike the bloodstream, which relies on the action of the heart for movement, the lymph system has no pump. Movement of muscles is required, which makes exercise of particular importance. Dry brushing also helps. It functions as a sort of lymph drainage massage.

It helps to break down cellulite deposits.
Seldom does one see an oriental woman with cellulite deposits on her hips. The reason? Dry brushing! It's considered an integral part of oriental

bathing practices. Cellulite is toxic material stored in the body's fat cells. Dry brushing helps to break down those deposits and flush them from the system.

It helps to improve blood circulation, plus the functioning of the brain, lungs, and heart.
Brushing the skin helps to relax muscles. When those in the chest are relaxed, lung function is improved. Consequently, blood quality is improved, and more oxygen is delivered to the brain and the heart.

HOW IS IT DONE?

The how-to's of dry brushing can be reduced to these three:

1. Always start at your extremities.
2. Always brush toward your heart. It's near that upper chest area on both sides of the sternum that the lymph system drains into the circulatory system.
3. Brush each segment of your body with at least seven strokes. Start lightly, especially on tender parts, and never brush so hard as to irritate the skin. From the back, come up and over the shoulders and around the neck.

It's best to brush before showering or doing colon cleansing. Brushing can be so invigorating to the body that doing so before bedtime may make it difficult to fall asleep. For some, however, just the opposite is true. Discover what works for you.

By the way, wash your brush every two weeks with soap and water.

Long-handled, natural bristle dry skin brushes can be found at most health food stores. They can also be ordered from Health*Quarters* Ministries. We carry a low-cost, high-quality brand. I have got two and I love them!

15

SOAKS AND SAUNAS

LIKE DRY BRUSHING, soaks and saunas are useful in supporting the health and detoxification function of the skin. Remember that your skin is the largest organ of detoxification. You need to sweat about two pounds of fluid a day.

Using the science of iridology (see chapter 30), you can look at your own eyes in a mirror and be able to tell if your skin is active or sluggish. If at the outer rim of your iris (the colored part of your eye) there is a darker ring around either part or all, that's a sign of underactive skin. You need to work at sweating more. Even if your skin appears to be fairly active, increasing your sweat is an important part of cleaning out your body.

It's a fact that most Americans simply do not sweat enough. We tend to wear tight or synthetic clothing that hinders the body's ability to breathe. We stop up our underarm sweat glands with gels, pastes, and powders. We force our lungs and kidneys to shoulder a bigger burden of waste products that should have been removed through our sweat. This taxes the organs' ability to function correctly.

Use of soaks (baths) and saunas on a regular basis to keep your skin open and active is important strategy in your overall cancer battle plan. Do these as often as possible. One or the other on a daily basis would be ideal.

SOAKS

The use of oil extracts from plants to stimulate the body's own cleansing and healing powers is called aromatherapy (see chapter 23). While this gives the impression of using these oils only as inhalants, they also do wonders when applied directly to the skin or used in baths.

Essential oils and products containing them are available in stores across the nation. Those manufactured by the network-marketing company Young Living are regarded by most in this field as superior in quality. Check your yellow pages for a Young Living Essential Oils distributor near you, or you may obtain a catalog and order directly from the company. To do so, you must give a sponsor's member number when you call them at 1-800-763-9963. If you wish, you may use Health*Quarters* Ministries as your sponsoring agent (member number 217162). You'll hear automated instructions. At their conclusion press 3 on your touch-tone phone to talk to a live operator. You'll be given your own member number to use from then on whenever you order.

Using Essential Oils in Soaks

- To de-stress, relax the nervous system, and create a feeling of overall well-being, choose from any of the following:

    Singles: chamomile, geranium, lavender, pine, birch, sandalwood, ylang ylang

    Blends: Gentle Baby, Harmony, Peace and Calming, Release

- To refresh, stimulate, and enhance the immune system, try:

    Singles: lemon, rosemary, thyme, peppermint, jasmine

    Blends: Awaken, Clarity, Envision

Special Instructions

- Use blends by themselves. Singles can be mixed.
- Use at least 3–5 drops for each soak.
- Adding a cup of Epsom salts can aid in muscle relaxing and help to pull toxins from the tissues.
- Adding extra drops of ginger oil will help to stimulate sweating.

- Make the water as hot as you can stand it without burning your skin. Soak for at least 30 minutes.

- DO NOT FORGET THE SOFT MUSIC AND CANDLELIGHT!

SAUNAS

- You want a dry heat sauna, not a steam room—unless the steam is made from purified water. Steam made from tap water will cause significant amounts of chlorine to be inhaled. (Ingestion of chlorinated water is associated with a 20 to 40 percent increase in the incidence of colon and rectal cancers.)[1] Asking your already overwhelmed liver to remove chlorine from your system is like shooting yourself in the foot when you're trying to win back and rebuild your health.

- It's wise to take a friend with you in case you get faint or lightheaded. If you've been having heart or circulatory problems (including high blood pressure), check with your doctor before doing saunas. If possible, take a plastic bottle of cold water into the sauna with you to sip from occasionally or to pour on your head now and then.

- Drink two to four glasses of water before entering.

- Dr. Keith Block suggests if you've been on chemo at any time in the recent past that you start with a low temperature and for about 10 to 15 minutes.[2] This, of course, assumes that you'll be able to control the temperature. Where I do my saunas, that's not possible. If that's true in your case, make your stay(s) shorter at first.

- Shower immediately to wash the toxins from your skin lest they be reabsorbed. I enjoy a regime where I do 10 minutes in the dry sauna, then a 30-second cold shower—repeating this three times, ending with cold. Enhancing blood flow through the system, it is a wonderful "kick in the proverbial butt" for the immune system.

- Take a liquid green drink after you're done to help replace minerals lost in sweat. I like the Kyo-Green powder for this.

16

REBOUNDING

IN PROFESSIONAL BASKETBALL a player who is a "rebounder" snags errant shots from backboards. This chapter, however, is about rebounding of a different sort. Referred to as a rebounder, the mini-trampoline is a key tool for helping to unload toxic wastes from our bodies. Using it, of course, is called rebounding.

LYMPH SYSTEM CLEANSER

The reason rebounding is such an effective form of detoxifying exercise has to do with its unique use of gravity. As a person bounces, the effects of gravitational force on the body change. "This force varies," explains Dr. Bruce Fife, "from zero Gs (one G is the earth's normal gravitational pull) at the top of the bounce, where the body is momentarily weightless, to as much as four Gs at the bottom of the bounce."[1] Four Gs means four times normal weight. A 120-pound woman would weigh 480 pounds. A 175-pound man would tip the scale at 700 pounds!

This variance in gravitational pull creates hydraulic pressure in the lymphatic system, helping to move lymph fluid filled with metabolic waste products toward its dumping site into the pulmonary bloodstream so that these wastes can eventually be removed from the body. Unlike the blood-stream, the lymph system has no pump and therefore relies on muscle movement and exercise to help it do its job.

The sorts of waste products that the lymph system is charged with removing from your body include things like dead and cancerous cells, nitrogenous wastes, fat, infectious viruses, heavy metals (aluminum, lead, mercury, etc.), and other assorted garbage.[2] One of the key weaknesses I find in a vast majority of folks I do nutritional assessments for is a sluggish lymph system. When the garbage disposal isn't working well, illness and disease are not far behind.

WHOLE BODY BUILDER

Helping to keep the lymph system doing its job of helping to detoxify the body is just one of the many benefits that come as a result of making rebounding a part of your daily exercise program. Here are more:

It strengthens all your muscles. Most forms of exercise work just a few of your many muscle groups. Rebounding, however, strengthens every muscle cell in the body as they respond to increased gravitational pull by becoming stronger. "In theory," says Dr. Fife, "rebounding at a force of two Gs (a relatively easy bounce) will double the strength of all body tissues. This includes all of the muscles, both skeletal and nonskeletal or involuntary muscles."[3]

It strengthens your heart. According to Dr. Morton Walker, rebounding is a key to heart health and function in two ways: "It improves the tone and quality of the muscles itself, and it increases the coordination of the fibers as they wring blood out of the heart during each beat."[4] Rebounding, he says, equals and often surpasses the aerobic effect of running but without the wear and tear on ankles, knees, and lower back.

It strengthens and stimulates bowel function. Your colon is a muscle. Its needs regular workouts to stay strong. Diets high in fiber give the colon muscle the resistance and bulk it needs to keep itself toned. Unfortunately, most Americans don't eat enough fiber. Our main pathway for removal of toxins is sluggish and weak. We are a nation of people who are chronically constipated.

Bottom line: rebounding strengthens every cell in your system. Every cell responds to the whole-body gravitational differences by becoming stronger. Your brain gets sharper. Your bones get harder. Your stomach digests food better. Your kidneys and liver purify blood and purge toxins better. And on and on. All this, and without the wear and tear on the body that so many other forms of exercise exact. Let me encourage you to make rebounding a daily pursuit, and for the rest of your life.

WHERE CAN I PURCHASE A REBOUNDER?

Most sporting goods stores carry them, even some department stores. Low end models start at about $30, with the high end reaching about $250. With a rebounder you get what you pay for. The cheaper they are, the more likely they are to suffer with use. Cheaper models tend to use low-quality springs that break more easily. I've been there, done that. I bought a cheap one at a department store once and was eventually sorry I did.

Needak Manufacturing makes the kind recommended by Dr. Walker. We use a Needak as part of the exercise program for the Health*Quarters* Lodge participants. It is not only top quality but also can be ordered with an attachable stabilizing bar to grasp while jumping.

Needak Manufacturing can be reached at 1-800-232-5762 or on the Internet at www.needakmfg.com.

HOW OFTEN SHOULD I USE IT?

The aggressiveness with which you approach rebounding depends on the physical condition in which you find yourself as you begin this new habit. If you're in the midst of trying to win back your health from some sort of degenerative disease process, it would be wise not only to start on the mild side, but to consult with your doctor before doing so. Gentle jumping, feet barely leaving the surface of the rebounder mat, is a great place to start. If you're in fairly good shape to begin with, a more aggressive jumping may be in order.

As far as how often to use your rebounder, I'd suggest daily—and in divided doses. Dr. Fife mentions that the effects of rebounding are cumulative. In other words, you don't need to do your entire workout all at once. Let me suggest you start with 5 minutes, three times daily. Of course, if you want to do all 15 minutes at once, go for it. Each week add another minute to each segment until you're doing 10 minutes three times a day.

FURTHER READING

The New Miracles of Rebound Exercise, by Albert E. Carter (Scottsdale, AZ: National Institute of Reboundology and Health), 1988.

17

PARASITE PURGING

PARASITES. Most Americans don't leave home without them!

You don't have to be a Third World traveler to find yourself the unwitting host to these unwelcome critters. You probably invite them in for dinner right there in your own home. Before I give you my strategy for purging parasites from your system, here is a summary of my discussion of parasites from chapter 6.

Potential Sizes *(once inside and fully developed)*

From one-celled, microscopic protozoa all the way up to 40-foot tapeworms

Potential Sources

Water (tap, mountain stream, well)

Pests (flies, fleas, cockroaches, mosquitoes)

Animals (dogs, cats, parakeets, livestock, beavers)

Foods (underwashed produce, undercooked meats)

Going barefoot in contaminated soils

Breathing dust (containing parasite eggs, cysts)

Close contact with others (day-care centers, sneezes, drinking from shared glasses, kissing, sexual intercourse, even just sharing a bed, shared toilet seats, sauna benches, whirlpools, bathtubs)

. . . and many, many more

The potential signs are as follows. The fact that these signs and symptoms can often be a signal of parasitical infestation does not necessarily mean that they always are. They also could be related to other causes. It is nevertheless wise to consider the possibility of parasites whenever faced with a disease process.

In Adults

Blue around lips
Puffy eyes
Persistent acne, skin eruptions, other skin problems
Heart palpitations
Blindness
Malabsorption of fat
Nutritional deficiencies (particularly vitamins A and B12)
Sinus congestion/heavy mucus
Gas and bloating
Cramps
Persistent bad breath
Teeth grinding during sleep
Intermittent loose/hard stools
Intestinal inflammation
Dysentery
Night sweats
Bloody stools
Ringing in the ears (tinnitus)
Anorexia
Chronic fatigue
Fluid retention (edema)
Hypoglycemic reactions
Depression
Nervousness
Weight gain

Painful urination
Foul-smelling, cheesy vaginal discharge
Swollen lymph glands
Seizures
Dark circles around eyes
Pale skin
Eye problems
Allergies (food/environmental)
Lactose intolerance
Lung/breathing problems
Abdominal distention
Severe dehydration
Sleep disturbances/insomnia
Intermittent diarrhea/constipation
Chronic constipation
Greasy stools
Flu-like symptoms (chills, fever)
Convulsions
Anal itching
Dizziness (vertigo)
Anemia
Joint/muscle pain
Sugar cravings
Disorientation/delusional behavior
Lethargy
Weight loss
Loss of appetite

Inflammation (prostate, bladder, vagina)

Paralysis on one side of the body

Migraine headaches

Parasites can generate symptoms often given the following labels: appendicitis, asthma, brain tumor, carcinoma, chronic fatigue syndrome, Crohn's disease, dermatitis, eczema, elephantiasis, encephalitis, epilepsy, fibromyalgia, gall bladder disease, hepatitis, Hodgkin's disease, irritable bowel syndrome, meningitis, mononucleosis, pneumonia, rheumatoid arthritis, schizophrenia, tinnitus, tuberculosis, ulcerative colitis

In Children (any of the preceding might apply, as well as these)

Dark circles under eyes

Grinding/clenching teeth during sleep

Constant nose picking or anal itching

Bed wetting

Unreasonable crying

Persistent limp

Night restlessness

Skin problems (rashes, eruptions)

Diagnosis of "failure to thrive" syndrome, celiac disease (distension of intestines and inability to absorb fats)

Hyperactivity

Dirt eating

Recurring headaches

Hair pulling (his or her own)

Convulsions

In Babies

Severe intermittent colic

Chronic crying

Head banging (against crib)

Anal rash

Does it seem like every major disease process is mentioned in these lists? Parasites are indeed at least a contributing factor to most of our health problems. Ninety-five percent of all Americans have them at any one time.

KILLING OFF UNWANTED GUESTS

Someone has said that house guests are like fish—after three days they begin to stink. If "stinking" was all that unwanted "internal" guests did, we'd all be in much better shape. Long-staying parasites that take up residence in our "innards," though, may well be the genesis of many disease processes.

How do you kill them off? Here is the Health*Quarters* 60-Day Parasite Purge plus ongoing maintenance plan.

Key sources from which the information on symptoms is taken include:

Guess What Came to Dinner, by Anne Louise Gittleman, M.S. (Avery, Garden City Park, NY, 1993)

Full of Life, by Luc De Schepper, M.D., Ph.D., Lic. Ac. (Tale Weaver, Los Angeles, 1991)

The Cure for All Cancers, by Hulda Regehr Clark, Ph.D., N.D. (ProMotion, San Diego, 1993)

HQ 60-DAY PARASITE PURGE

Days 1–10: *Improve Digestion*
Tools: Food enzymes and B-complex vitamins

Many parasites enter our bodies by way of food and drink. If the stomach is producing adequate amounts of hydrochloric acid (HCl), they are usually destroyed before they can take up residence and multiply. However, as we age we tend to produce less and less HCl. This is compounded by the fact that sugar, caffeine, and dairy products tend to rob the body of B-complex vitamins, which are used to manufacture HCl.

Food enzymes from Nature's Sunshine is a product I like to give my clients that assists digestion by providing HCl along with certain digestive enzymes. A typical dose is two to three with each meal.

B-vitamins are also important to replenish the body's stores and facilitate production of its own digestive acids. A typical amount is 100 mg per day.

Improve Elimination
Tools: Fiber and marshmallow/pepsin

The intestinal tract is a key hiding place for many parasites. The way we typically tend to eat as Americans leads to the buildup of encrusted fecal matter and rubbery mucus along the intestinal wall, forming a hose within a hose. Between the false lining that has been formed and the real lining of the intestine, "critters," yeasts, and all manner of other "nasties" tend to make their home.

Fiber works as an intestinal broom and detoxifying agent to sweep and cleanse the walls of the intestinal tract. The typical dose I suggest is 1 teaspoon mixed in 8 ounces of water upon rising, another teaspoon one-half hour before lunch, and a third before bedtime. Be sure to drink lots of purified water throughout the day. The hydration formula is as given in chapter 10: divide your body weight in half, calling that ounces. Divide that number by 8, and you get the number of 8-ounce glasses a day you should consume.

Marshmallow/pepsin combination is a second product I give to help clean out the intestinal tract. Pockets can form in the intestinal wall that fiber products can't clean out. They become a haven for putrifying waste products and parasites. Marshmallow is a sticky herb. It sticks the pepsin, a digestive enzyme, to the intestinal wall, allowing it to "digest" the debris and parasites out of the pockets. The suggested dose is two with each meal.

Days 11–60: Send in the Killers

Tool: Chinese Para-Cleanse

Keep taking the Day 1–10 products until the bottles are empty.

Chinese Para-Cleanse is an herbal blend of pumpkin seeds, black walnut hulls, casgara sagrada bark, violet leaf, chamomile flowers, mullein leaves, marshmallow root, slippery elm bark, caprylic acid, red raspberry leaves, elecampane root and bark, spearmint leaf, turmeric root, garlic bulb, ginger root, and clove bud. These herbs work together as a team to weaken and destroy parasites in the system.

To use this product effectively, three bags must be used. Each bag contains 20 smaller bags, each containing six capsules. Each morning 15 minutes before breakfast, take the capsules in one of the small bags. Each evening 15 minutes before dinner, take another small bag. Do this for 10 days. You will have finished the contents of an entire large bag. Lay off for 10 days, then do another 10-day round. Lay off for another 10 days, finishing with a final 10-day round. (The lay-off periods are to allow time for eggs to hatch so that they may be more readily destroyed.)

ONGOING MAINTENANCE

Tool: *Super 7*

Because we live in a world in which we're daily exposed to potential sources of parasitical infection, keeping the body strong against them is of vital importance. *Super 7* is a grouping of seven key products I drew together to help keep your blood, internal organs, and tissues cleansed, well nourished, and strong. Look for these products at your local health food store or order them from Health*Quarters.* They include:

1. New Image Total—a powerful blend of antioxidants to protect against the damaging effects of free radicals.

2. New Image Plus—a blend of chromium picolinate and herbs that helps to regulate blood sugar, energy, and the buildup of lean muscle tissue.

3. New Image Cleanse and

4. Encapsulated Psyllium Seeds—two products that help to clean and tone the bowel.

5. Supper Supplemental without iron—a blend of vitamins and minerals used to help augment those derived from dietary sources.

Additional Thoughts

- When one person in a family has a parasitical infection, it's a safe bet that all do. All family members living together under one roof should undertake parasite cleansing at the same time.

- Get your pets de-wormed regularly.

- Drink only purified water. Get yourself a home water purifier. And if you're on well rather than city water, don't assume it's clean just because it comes from a well. Again, drink no water unless it's been purified. *Giardia* (microscopic organisms) are notorious for being found in well water.

6. Friendly flora to help repopulate the intestinal tract.

7. Food Enzymes—a blend of hydrochloric acid and digestive enzymes to help ensure good digestion and nutrient absorption.

Many of the items listed in this chapter may be available at your local health food store or nutritional consultant. They are also available from Health-*Quarters* Ministries.

18

JUICE FASTING AND COLON/LIVER CLEANSING

FASTING FOR THE HEALTH OF IT means to abstain from solid foods for a time in order to allow the body to focus its energies on cleansing and healing, instead of digestion. Digestion, particularly of concentrated protein foods, is the hardest work our internal organs are asked to do. The fruit and vegetable juices used in juice fasting require little to no digestive energies from the body yet are loaded with the nutrients, enzymes, and alkalinizing agents that our various organs and systems require to maintain health while cleansing and healing.

An integral part of juice fasting involves colon and liver cleansing via water and coffee enemas. When people attend the Health*Quarters* Lodge to go through an 11-day "detox and lifestyle change" session, many of the health benefits they derive from their stay are a result of this fasting-cleansing combination. Otto Buchinger, Jr., M.D., considered by many the greatest fasting authority in the world, calls juice fasting a "royal road to healing."

QUESTIONS MOST OFTEN ASKED ABOUT
THE JUICE-FASTING PROCESS

How Do I Make Juice?

You're going to need a good juicer. I recommend the Champion as the best for the money. It is noted for maintaining a better supply of enzymes than other juicers. It can even be purchased with an attachment that allows for milling grain into flour. You might be able to find a Champion for sale at your local health food store. They are also available from Health*Quarters*.

Use only organically grown produce if at all possible. Whether organic or not, soak it for 15 minutes in a sink of water containing a cup of hydrogen peroxide. This will help remove parasites, bacteria, and any chemical residues from the skin.

When making a juice of fruits or veggies, add 6 ounces fresh juice to 4 ounces purified water. Too much natural sugar from juice can be hard on the pancreas. A cookbook I wrote called *Raw, Raw, Raw* will give you ideas for juice combinations. The only fruits you can juice together with veggies are apples and lemons. Aside from these two, fruit and vegetable juices should never be mixed.

Fresh juices will lose most of their enzymes within about 30 minutes if allowed to remain exposed to air. Either drink them immediately or store them in vacuum-sealed thermoses. They'll keep for about eight hours.

Are There Specific Juices I Should Emphasize?

- *Apple juice* helps purify and alkalinize the blood, clean the bladder, ward off intestinal infections, reduce inflammation of the colon, reduce blood cholesterol, stabilize blood sugar, reduce appetite, reduce blood pressure, detoxify heavy metals from the system, protect against damage from X-rays and radiation therapy, and inhibit cancer cells.

- *Beet juice* helps build red blood cells, protect against anemia, stimulate digestion, eliminate the buildup of acid materials in the bowel, reduce cholesterol, aid the lymphatic system, protect the liver and gallbladder, and inhibit cancer cells.

- *Carrot juice* helps reduce blood cholesterol, relieve constipation and other colon disorders, support skin and tissue health, boost the immune system, and prevent heart and circulatory diseases. Studies show that the beta-carotene in carrot juice helps to inhibit cancer cells by disrupting the mechanism that initially turns good cells into bad.

- *Celery juice* helps to alkalinize the bloodstream, purify the blood, improve digestion, aid kidney and liver function, enhance the activity of white blood cells, halt fermentation, and inhibit cancer cells. Organic sodium is known as the "youth element" helping to keep the body youthful and limber. Celery is loaded with it.

- *Cabbage juice.* Studies show that the cabbage family of vegetables (also known as cruciferous) contains more known anticancer properties than any other grouping. Included in this family, besides various kinds of cabbage are broccoli, Brussels sprouts, cauliflower, watercress, horseradish, kale, kohlrabi, mustard greens, radish, rutabaga, and turnip.

Why Is It Necessary to Do Enemas While Juice Fasting?

During a juice fast the body expends little energy on metabolism, allowing it to focus on cleansing and healing. It will take the opportunity to burn diseased tissues and dead cells, as well as to dump toxic wastes into the bloodstream that may have been accumulating in the system for years. These toxic wastes can be purged from the body through any of four paths—the skin, lungs, kidneys, bowel—with the bowel being the main highway.

Enemas are used to help ensure that toxic wastes are regularly and often leaving the body via the bowel. Without their use, toxins are easily reabsorbed through the colon wall into the bloodstream, poisoning the whole system. This is referred to as autointoxication.

Note: Some health care professionals consider enemas a controversial issue. Please bear in mind that what I'm presenting here are concepts and possibilities, not prescriptions. Juice fasting in conjunction with colon plus liver cleaning via enemas has proven itself helpful in many, many situations. However, this information is not meant to replace the advice of a professional health care practitioner of your choice, fully aware of your unique situation. Before making any application of this information, it would be in your best interest to seek out such advice.

What's the Purpose of Coffee Enemas?

Coffee enemas are called retention enemas, for the objective is to hold the fluid in the lower part of the colon (sigmoid) for about 20 minutes. Caffeine is absorbed through the intestinal wall into the bloodstream and deliv-

> **Frähm's Principle of Juice Fasting**
>
> Make friends with your water and coffee enemas.

ered directly to the liver by way of a hepatic vein, thereby providing stimulation for the liver to purge and cleanse itself. (The coffee does not go through the digestive system.)

Simply drinking coffee does not render the same liver-purging effect. As discussed in chapter 3, "Toxic Diet," caffeine introduced through the digestive system can be a burden to the body's ability to maintain health. To make a point of the potential value of coffee enemas, here are the thoughts of many well-respected health care professionals. Again, let me remind you that this is a concept and a possibility to explore, not a prescription for your particular situation.

SHERRY A. ROGERS, M.D.

The coffee enema has saved many lives. A coffee what? An enema? With what? How gross! How weird! How sordid! You mean you stick it in your butt?? How disgusting! But on the contrary, how healing and how life saving. And for some it is the difference between life and death.

A coffee enema could save the day for . . . victims of overwhelming toxicity. As we have found, they are invaluable in numerous conditions, from postoperative healing, severe infections, severe and traumatic injuries, to speeding the recovery time from chemical exposures and cancers.[1]

PATRICK QUILLIN, PH.D., R.D.

Enemas are one of the oldest healing modalities in human literature. . . . Coffee enemas have been in the Merck Medical Manual for decades until 1977, when editors of the manual claimed that this revered therapy was eliminated for "lack of space" in the new manuscript. The reality is that coffee enemas became the focal point in criticizing alternative cancer therapies.[2]

JAMES F. BALCH, M.D., AND PHYLLIS A. BALCH, C.N.C.

Coffee used in this way has a different effect on the body than if it were ingested orally. When used in an enema, it does not go through the normal digestion process. It is beneficial in treatment when used properly because it stimulates the liver to excrete toxins or "poison bile." . . . As well as treatment for liver toxins, coffee enemas are used while fasting to relieve headaches caused by the buildup of toxins during detoxification.[3]

MAX GERSON, M.D.

Inasmuch as the detoxification of the body is of the greatest importance, especially in the beginning, it is absolutely necessary to administer frequent enemas. . . . Coffee enemas are not given for the function of the intestines, but for the stimulation of the liver. . . . The effect is an increased production of bile, an opening of the bile ducts, and greater flow of bile.[4]

Linda Rector Page, N.D., Ph.D.

Coffee enemas have become standard in natural healing when liver- and blood-related cancers are present. Caffeine used in this way stimulates the liver and gallbladder to remove toxins, open bile ducts, encourage increased peristaltic action, and produce necessary enzyme activity for healthy red blood cell formation and oxygen uptake.[5]

Won't Enemas Make Me Dependent on Them for Bowel Movements?

It's the fiber in one's diet that not only sweeps the intestinal tract clean of toxic debris but also creates bulk for the colon muscle to push against. In this way the colon stays toned and strong, able to push waste through. Conversely, it's the lack of fiber in the typical American's diet that leads many to have a flabby, underactive intestinal tract.

Water, as in water enemas, can have the same toning effect on the colon, giving it something to push against. There are many in the field of natural health who claim that instead of making one dependent on them for bowel movements, enemas actually help to strengthen the peristaltic action of the bowel for better and more frequent bowel movements once enemas are removed from the daily agenda.

How Are Enemas Done?

Enema kits can be purchased from most drugstores, and from Health-*Quarters*.

Water Enemas

Warm up 4 quarts of purified water (distilled or reverse osmosis—do NOT use tap water). Fill the hot water bottle in the enema kit (2 quarts), making sure air is squeezed out before screwing in the tube. Allow a bit of water through the tube so it is full before closing the clamp. This way you won't be allowing air into your colon when you administer the enema. Not life-threatening if you do, just a little uncomfortable.

Lay a towel on your bathroom floor. Lubricate your enema tip with olive or vitamin E oil (don't use Vaseline, since petroleum products are not good to have on your skin). A product called Un-Petroleum Jelly found in most health food stores could also be used.

Hook the enema bag over the bathroom doorknob, or you might wish to hang it from a towel rack. In any case, you want to have the bag at least 12–24 inches higher than your body.

Lie down on your left side and gently insert your lubricated enema tip. Gradually release the water. When you begin to feel a sensation of fullness or an urge to release, clamp the water flow and wait a bit. If the urge to release passes, open the clamp and continue to fill your colon. If it doesn't pass, remove the tip and evacuate your bowel, then start the process once again.

After each time you fill your colon, massage your abdomen up the left side, across, and down the right. After each time you evacuate, massage up the right side, across, and down the left. If you're unable to take in a full bag at a time, don't fret. Do as much as you can, trying to do more each time. Do a total of four quarts of purified water (two full bags) during each water enema session.

Coffee Retention Enemas

Brew 2–3 cups of water with 4 tablespoons of organically grown coffee, adding 1–2 cups of cool water to get a lukewarm water temperature. Lie on your left side to insert the tip, and release 4 cups of fluid. Hold the fluid in your colon for 15–20 minutes. When evacuating, if nothing comes out, don't worry. You've absorbed the fluid.

If you experience difficulty retaining the coffee, add 1 tablespoon of Epsom salts to the brew before inserting. This is magnesium, a muscle relaxant. If you're experiencing problems with the water enema, try adding 1 tablespoon of Epsom salts to each bag.

Cleaning Your Enema Tools

When you're done, rinse all parts with hot water. Wipe the lubricant tip and store it in a small glass bottle of Clorox bleach. Storing your bag and tube in a large Ziplock bag is a good idea.

Additional Comments

- ALWAYS use organically grown coffee. You can purchase cans through Health*Quarters* or from your health food store. Even some mainline supermarkets are now carrying organic coffee. If you use conventionally grown, you're going to be putting pesticide residues into the system you're trying to detoxify.

- ALWAYS use caffeinated coffee. The caffeine stimulates your liver.

- NEVER use instant coffee.

- I've shared the details of the way I do enemas. Other teachers will have different details. Do what works for you.

- Once you get the hang of coffee enemas, you'll find them both relaxing and energizing. (As you're detoxing, they may also be a bit nauseating.)

- During a fast, do two water and two coffee enemas a day. The rest of the month do one water and one coffee enema. See the "game plan" at the end of this chapter.

Will I Lose a Lot of Weight on a Juice Fast?

We have folks from both sides of the coin come spend sessions with us at our Lodge. Some want to shed some pounds. Others don't. What I have noted through my experience is that the body involved in juice fasting tends to lose weight to where it wants to be, then maintains that level.

Most folks going through a seven-day juice fast tend to lose some weight. Some of this is water weight, as the inflammation from a typical array of food allergies begins to be diminished in the cleansing/healing system. In addition, as mucus ropes and hardened fecal matter are washed from the intestinal tract, weight can be dropped. It has been estimated that the average American tends to be carrying around 7 to 60 pounds of such material in his or her "gut."

There are situations where fasting is inappropriate. In some advanced disease situations where the body has entered what might be termed a wasting process, fasting is contraindicated. Fat reserves are gone, and the body is feeding on muscle tissues. In these cases the objective, instead of cleansing, is building. The individual should be feasting—but on foods that are health promoting, easily digested, and help to build reserves—not milkshakes and beefsteaks. Chapter 19, "The 80/20 Diet," should be helpful here.

Will My Vital Organs Be Weakened in Any Way?

My best answer to this one comes from the observations of Paavo Airola, Ph.D., N.D, a very big name in the field of nutrition and natural health. Here's what he has to say in his book *How to Get Well:*

> During the prolonged fast (after the first three days), your body will live on its own substance . . . it will burn and digest its own tissues by the process of autolysis, or self-digestion. But, your body will not do it indiscriminately! In its wisdom—and here lies the secret of the extraordinary

effectiveness of fasting as curative and rejuvenate therapy—your body will first decompose and burn those cells and tissues which are diseased, damaged, aged or dead. In fasting, your body feeds itself on the most impure and inferior materials, such as dead cells and morbid accumulations, tumors, abscesses, fat deposits, etc. . . . The essential tissues and vital organs, the glands, the nervous system and the brain are not damaged or digested in fasting.[6]

Will I Get Too Hungry?

I've personally experienced, and observed of others, that the fires of hunger are more than adequately doused when multiple juices, supplements, herbal teas, and glasses of water are taken daily.

The most common statement heard during nutrition classes is, "I can't believe I've gone this many days and I'm still not hungry." The first three days can be touchy for some. Frequent consumption of juices and fiber keep the hunger down, but folks miss the activity of eating and chewing. Usually by day 4 most are over that hump. Some, when day 7 rolls around and it's time to break the fast, chose not to. That's fine. Some "kick butt" nutritionists will put people on 14-day juice fasts right off the bat, especially if they're fighting an aggressive disease process. They are, of course, not treating the disease but using fasting to direct the body's energies toward cleansing and healing.

Bottom line: hunger on a juice fast is usually more a state of mind than a condition of the stomach. That is, if you're doing enough fluids and fiber.

What Might I Expect to Be Happening in My Body?

This rule will not always be the case, and in fact one day on a fast may be different from the next, depending on what the body is doing internally. I've witnessed people "lower than a duck's instep" one day and flying off the walls with new energy the next.

The detoxification process is not a picnic in the park. The body is engaged in intense work, pulling toxic buildup and waste products "out of storage" throughout the system—from fat, muscles, tissues, and organs. Initiating a fast, you send the signal to your system that it has the freedom to dump. Garbage will be thrown out into the bloodstream for eventual removal, and this can lead to what is commonly termed a healing crisis.

In my studies I ran across the following list of what to be ready for

---

Frähm's Principle of Juice Fasting

Expect to feel worse before you feel better. Let me repeat that. EXPECT TO FEEL WORSE BEFORE YOU FEEL BETTER!

while undertaking a fast. I can't give credit to its author, unfortunately, having lost that information. But I can say that I've witnessed most of these types of things happening in people during juice fasting at our Lodge.

Discomforts may include any or all of the following:

Fatigue	Soft stools
Increased need for sleep	Loss of memory
Insomnia	Loss of motivation
Skin rashes and eruptions	Nausea
Nervousness	Dizziness
Panic attacks	Hypoglycemia-like reactions
Headaches	Depression, anger, anxiety
Nightmares	Bad breath
Lack of concentration	Foul body odor
Irritability	Symptoms of past illnesses

As toxins are filtered out of the circulation processes into the excretory organs, the body will select the most convenient route of excretion available to it. These may include:

- Kidneys (dark urine with bad odor)

- Colon (runny stools, mucus ropes, smelly)

- Skin (smelly sweat, foul body odor, eruptions)

- Nose (runny)

- Eyes (watery, blurry)

- Lungs (bad breath, phlegm)

As "internal house cleaning" progresses, you may experience any or all of the following:

- Increased energy and vitality

- Clearer thinking

- Increased ability to handle stress

- Increased resistance to colds and flu

- Enhanced feelings of well-being (physical, mental, emotional)

- Reduced cancer count

- Disappearance of allergies

To aid your detox process, avoid the following:

- Medications to suppress symptoms
- All animal products
- Emotional stress

Should I Be Taking Supplements While Doing a Juice Fast?

Yes. It has been estimated that it takes five to seven times the amount of nutrients to regain one's health as it does to simply maintain it. Taking a few strategic supplements along with freshly made juices helps to flood the body with easily utilized nutrients for cleansing and healing, while at the same time allowing the liver and digestive tract to take a break from the digestive process.

Here's a list of supplements we use during the fasting program. Check for them at your local health food store or through your health care professional. They are also available from Health*Quarters*.

Blood Cleansers

- *Essiac tea* (I prefer a product called E-Tea capsules). A blend of burdock root, sheep sorrel herb, slippery elm bark, and Turkey rhubarb root. These herbs work synergistically to purify the blood, clean the liver/gallbladder, bind up toxins in the bowel, and stimulate the immune system. Two capsules can be opened into hot water to make tea.

- *Green drink* (I prefer a product called Kyo-Green powder). A blend of barley grass and wheat grass powders, Bulgaria chlorella, cooked brown rice, and Pacific kelp. Grasses, chlorella, and kelp contain chlorophyll, which is considered the best cleansing and purifying agent in nature. It stops bacteria growth in the digestive system, deodorizes the body, removes drug deposits and toxins from cells, detoxifies the kidneys and liver, deactivates manmade carcinogens, builds and enriches the blood, renews and strengthens intestines, improves liver function, and activates enzymes to produce vitamins A, E, and K.

    Chlorella in particular binds with heavy metals, pesticides, and other carcinogens and carries them from the body, stimulates interferon production and other antitumor and immune-enhancing activity, protects against mutations, and contains nucleic acid (RNA/DNA), which directs the renewal, growth, and repair of cells.

Kelp is a rich source of vitamins, particularly Bs, plus minerals and trace elements. Kelp also contains an abundance of organic iodine, which is food for the thyroid gland.

Liver Cleansers

- *LIV-A (capsules)*. A blend of herbs historically used to nourish the liver. Contains red beet root, dandelion root, parsley herb, horsetail herb, yellow dock root, black cohosh root, birch leaves, blessed thistle herb, angelica root, chamomile flowers, gentian root, and goldenrod herb.

- *UltraClear Plus (powder)*. Designed to support nutritional needs during liver detoxification. Contains beta-carotene, biotin, calcium, carbhydrate, chromium, copper, fiber, folic acid, iodine, L-cysteine, L-glutathione, magnesium, manganese, N-acetylcysteine, niacinamide, B5, phosphorus, organic iron, potassium, protein, and other nutrients.

Colon Cleansers

- *Fiber.* I like a product called Perfect 7 powder, a blend of psyllium seed, psyllium husks, milk-free lactobacillus bifidus powder, bentonite, alfalfa leaf, cascara sagrada bark, rose hips, buckthorn bark, capsicum, garlic, and goldenseal. Helps provide bulk to the stool in order to stimulate bowel action and to clean and tone the lining of the small and large intestines.

- *Flora.* I like a product called PB8 capsules, a dairy-free probiotic designed to help repopulate the intestinal tract with healthy bacteria. It contains eight different strains of "friendly flora" microorganisms that naturally inhabit the intestinal tract. They aid digestion and absorption of nutrients, and they enhance immune function.

- *Aloe vera* (I like a product called New Image Cleanse tablets). Helps kill pathogenic bacteria, viruses, yeasts, and parasites. Neutralizes damage from radiation and chemotherapy. Reduces inflammation. Helps remove tumors, growths, dead cells, and toxic substances. Cleanses and heals tissues. Stimulates bowel action.

Key Nutrients

- *Vitamin C with bioflavonoids* (I like a product called Super C powder). Stimulates the immune system to produce interferon, an antitumor chemical. Helps wounded tissues heal. It is a highly effective natural chelator for binding up pesticide residues and heavy metals (mercury, lead, aluminum, etc.) and flushing them from the body. Its power is made twice as potent when taken with bioflavonoids.

- *Proanthocyanidins*. I like a product called New Image Total capsules, a blend of pine bark and grape seed extracts (each 50 times more powerful than vitamin E and 20 times more powerful than vitamin C), plus quercetin from blue-green algae, vitamin C, Siberian ginseng, zinc picolinate, vitamin B6, ginkgo biloba, L-cysteine, silymarin (milk thistle extract), selenium, vitamin E, and beta-carotene. Helps to cleanse and protect the body from free radicals, inflammation processes, bacterial infections, cholesterol deposits, liver toxicities, and heavy metals.

- *Bromelain (capsules)*. A protein-digestive enzyme derived from pineapple, it is useful for the digestion of "foreign" protein in the body. Parasites and cancer cells are such proteins.

How Long Should Juice Fasts Be, and How Often Should I Do Them?

I suggest a three-day juice fast for simply purging the body of toxins and cleaning up the blood. Making this a monthly habit would be good for all. For those winning back their health from a disease process, I suggest a seven-day juice fast once a month until health is regained. James Balch, M.D., observes that after five days the healing and rebuilding of the immune system starts.[7] I've noted with our Lodge participants that seven days seems just right—long enough to stimulate good cleansing and healing yet short enough to feel doable.

What Should I Eat and What Supplements Should I Take When I'm Not Fasting?

I like to suggest a plant-based diet composed of about 80 percent raw foods (see chapter 19). I also suggest the following during those weeks:

- One water and one coffee enema each day

- Four fresh juices each day

- The ten fasting supplements each day

- In addition, include the following supplements in your daily agenda:

Digestion Builders

- *B-complex*. The stomach uses B-vitamins to help produce hydrochloric acid. This is necessary for the proper digestion of fats and proteins.

Sugar, caffeine, dairy products, and stress rob the body of its stores of B. Replenishing your supply of Bs is of vital importance.

- *Betaine hydrochloride* (hydrochloric acid)

- *Digestive enzymes.* Four things must be present in the stomach in order for proper digestion to take place: flora, B-vitamins, hydrochloric acid, and digestive enzymes. To supply the latter two I like a product called Food Enzymes—a combination of hydrochloric acid and enzymes.

Immune System Builders

- *Cat's claw,* also known as *uña de gato* (I like a product called Cat's Claw Combination that contains cat's claw, astragalus, and echinacea). Studies have shown that this herb helps to counteract the side effects of chemotherapy and radiation. European and South American researchers have noted its significant effectiveness at inhibiting cancer cells. Its ability to strengthen the immune system is remarkable.

- *Astragalus.* Studies show that this herb helps to improve energy, halt "wasting" conditions, and improve the immune system. It has been used in traditional Chinese medicine for thousands of years and is currently being reviewed by the American Cancer Society because of its observed benefit to the immune system of people fighting cancer.

- *Echinacea.* A well-known and highly prized immune system strengthener, as well as blood and lymph system cleanser.

Include as well the cell builder *flaxseed oil* (I like a product called Barlean's liquid). It provides the body with a rich supply of essential fatty acids (EFAs). These are not produced by the body but must come from the diet. They are necessary for the production of prostaglandins—substances that regulate all cellular functions and structure.

The charts below should assist you in planning your fast.

Monthly Overview (daily amounts; t = tsp; T = tbsp; caps = capsules)		
	Fasting	**80/20 Diet**
Essiac tea (E-tea)	2 caps, 3x	2 caps, 2x
Apple juice	2 glasses	2 glasses
Vegetable juice	3 glasses	2 glasses
UltraClear Plus	2 scoops, 3x	———
Green drink (Kyo-Green)	1 t, 3x	1 t, 2x

Monthly Overview (daily amounts) (continued)

	Fasting	80/20 Diet
LIV-A	2 caps, 3x	2 caps, 3x
Fiber (Perfect 7)	1 t, 3x	1 t, 2x
Flora (PB8)	4 caps, 1x	4 caps, 1x
Aloe vera (New Image Total)	2 tab, 1x	2 tab, 1x
Vitamin C w bioflavonoids (Super C)	1 t, 3x	1 t, 3x
Proanthocyanidins (New Image Total)	1 cap per 25 lbs	2 caps, 1x
Bromelain (on empty stomach)	5 caps, 3x	3 caps, 2x
B-vitamins	——	1 cap, 3x
Food enzymes	——	2 tabs each meal
Cat's claw combination	——	1 cap, 3x
Flaxseed oil	——	1 T, 3x

Water enemas	2x/day	1x/day
Coffee enemas	2x/day	1x/day
Soaks or saunas	3/week	3/week
Dry brush	1x/day	1x/day
Liver/gallbladder flush	1x/per fast	——
Deep breathing	1 min, 3x/day	1 min, 3x/day
Rebounding	5 min, 1x/day	15 min, 1x/day
Walking	15 min, 1x/day	30 min, 1x/day

Sample 7-Day Juice Fasting Schedule (Assuming an 8 to 5 workday)

Time	Juice and Supplements	Activities
6:00 a.m.	E-tea	Make juices and put in thermos for work
6:30 a.m.	UltraClear Plus + LIV-A + Total	Dry brush + enemas (water and coffee)
8:30 a.m.	Bromelain	
9:00 a.m.	Veggie juice + Kyo-Green + vit C	Deep breathing
10:00 a.m.	Apple juice + Perfect 7	
11:00 a.m.	Veggie juice + Kyo-Green + vit C	

Sample 7-Day Juice Fasting Schedule (Assuming an 8 to 5 workday)		
Time	**Juice and Supplements**	**Activities**
Noon	UltraClear Plus + LIV-A + Total	Deep breathing
1:00 p.m.	Bromelain	
2:00 p.m.	E-tea	
3:00 p.m.	Veggie juice + Kyo-Green + vit C	Deep breathing
4:00 p.m.	Apple juice + Perfect 7	
6:00 p.m.	UltraClear Plus + LIV-A + Total	
7:00 p.m.	Bromelain	Exercise
8:00 p.m.	E-tea	
9:00 p.m.	Perfect 7 + New Image Cleanse	Enema (water)
9:30 p.m.		Soak or sauna
10:00 p.m.	Bedtime + PB8	

Since this example is built around a work schedule, the second coffee enema of the day will be hard to accomplish. Doing one too late in the day (after work, in other words) may disrupt your sleep. Add a midday coffee enema on weekends. On the evening of day 3 of the fast, do the liver/gallbladder flush just before bed (see the instructions in chapter 12).

Sample 80/20 Diet Schedule (Assuming an 8 to 5 workday)		
Time	**Juice and Supplements**	**Activities**
6:00 a.m.	E-tea	Make juices and put in thermos for work
6:30 a.m.	Apple juice & Perfect 7	Dry brush + Enemas (water and coffee)
7:30 a.m.	Breakfast . . . LIV-A + vit C + Total + B-complex + food enzymes + cat's claw comb. + flaxseed oil	
9:00 a.m.	Bromelain	Deep breathing
10:30 a.m.	Veggie juice + Kyo-Green	
Noon	Lunch . . . LIV-A + vit C + B-complex + food enzymes + cat's claw comb. + flaxseed oil	

Sample 80/20 Diet Schedule (Assuming an 8 to 5 workday)		
Time	**Juice and Supplements**	**Activities**
2:00 p.m.	Bromelain	Deep breathing
3:00 p.m.	Veggie juice + Kyo-Green	
6:00 p.m.	Dinner . . . LIV-A + vit C + B-complex + food enzymes + cat's claw comb. + flaxseed oil	
7:00 p.m.		Exercise and deep breathing
8:00 p.m.	Apple juice + Perfect 7 + New Image Cleanse	
9:00 p.m.		Soak or sauna
10:00 p.m.	Bedtime + PB8	

Note: If you are serious about making juicing and juice fasting a part of your own cancer battle plan but don't find all the answers here you're looking for, let me encourage you to give us a call. You'll find the Health*Quarters* phone number listed in appendix A. You might want to consider taking part in our 11-day Lodge sessions. It's a great way to get a solid start toward renewed health.

Short of attending the Lodge, seek out the advice of a professional health care provider near you who is familiar with your unique needs. Do this before making application of this "fasting/cleansing" information to your own situation. If you need help locating professional help that comes from the same general "camp" that Health*Quarters* Ministries does, order a copy of our Health Resources List.

TOOLS FOR STRENGTHENING

Our body was made to be well. Its constant desire and continuous effort is always geared toward being well. Should it not be well, it has an amazing capacity to restore and even heal itself.

With such a force on our side, it should be unusual for us to be ill, and in fact, it is true that disease and sickness are abnormal. Therefore, it follows that if we would fully cooperate and join forces with our bodies, sickness should rarely occur.

ALBERT ZEHR, PH.D., *Healthy Steps*

YOU'VE EXAMINED the "rocks." You've learned ways and means to clean out your body and your mind. Now it's time to talk a little "body building" and learn to join forces with your body to help restore its potent self-protective and self-healing powers.

19

THE 80/20 DIET

WHEN FOLKS COME to our Lodge to learn the principles of nutrition that will help them win back their health, I teach them our Health*Quarters* 80/20 diet. It's a primarily raw foods diet—80 percent raw, 20 percent cooked.

Why raw? In a word, enzymes. Raw foods have them. Cooked foods don't. Imagine your car without its spark plugs. Enzymes are the most studied phenomena of the human body, yet most of us are completely unaware of their existence, let alone knowing what they do for us. Every system, every process, every chemical reaction in our bodies is initiated and carried out by enzymatic activity.

Scientists have identified thousands upon thousands of different types of enzymes that function in the body, with billions of each type doing their unique work. They supervise and run our immune system, bloodstream, liver, kidneys, digestive system, heart, spleen, pancreas—you name it. Even our abilities to see, think, and breathe depend on enzymes.

YOUR ENZYME BANK ACCOUNT

There are two broad categories of enzymes in this world: (1) metabolic enzymes (also known as body enzymes), manufactured in the bodies of living things, and (2) food enzymes (also known as plant enzymes), obviously found in plants.

Three things are true about these wonders of creation that are important to anyone who wishes to be the best caretaker of his or her body that he or she can be:

1. The metabolic enzymes that keep our bodies functioning are continually being used up, needing to be replenished on a regular basis.

2. Our bodies require live enzymes from an outside source, which they then transform into the various kinds of metabolic enzymes needed.

3. The only outside source for live enzymes are raw foods or special enzyme supplements carefully manufactured from raw food sources. Cooking or otherwise processing a food destroys its enzymes.

Each of us is endowed with a limited enzyme reserve at birth. A diet high in cooked or processed foods is a continual drain on that account. Your body is actually being robbed every time you eat cooked foods. Unless your enzyme account receives steady deposits, sooner than expected your funds will dry up.

Don't get into the habit of relying heavily on enzyme supplements in place of making raw foods a lifestyle. The most important thing you can do for your health is to eat a diet high in raw produce (fruits, veggies, grains, seeds, and nuts). Of course, skip the raw fish and meat.

ALKALINIZE OR DIE!

A second important reason for eating a diet consisting primarily of raw fruits and vegetables has to do with our body's need for alkalinity. The human body functions best when our blood is slightly alkaline. We make acid as a natural by-product of metabolism, but we make no alkaline. We must therefore get alkalinizing minerals from our diets. All foods burn down, after digestion, into either acid or alkaline ash. Whereas most cooked foods burn to acid in the body, most raw fruits and veggies burn to alkaline.

Joel Robbins, M.D., of Tulsa, Oklahoma, uses the example of a young calf to underscore the importance of enzyme replacement. He points out that if you apply enough heat to cow's milk to kill all its enzymes (at 112 degrees they begin to die), and feed it back to a calf as its only food, the calf will die within a couple of months.[1]

In addition, acidic conditions are the forerunner of degenerative diseases, and they leave the body susceptible to parasites. A body that is slightly alkaline will destroy microscopic invaders from the outside world. However, a body that has regressed into a chronic, acidic state because of a diet made up primarily of cooked and/or heat-processed foods will be highly susceptible to parasitic activity.

NUTRIENTS AND FIBER

Two additional benefits of eating the 80/20 diet are nutrients and fiber. When food is cooked, nutrients are destroyed—a topic addressed in more detail in chapter 3.

Concerning fiber—plants have it, animals don't. There is no fiber in any meat or dairy product. And yet fiber is essential for keeping waste products from getting congested in our intestinal tract and, eventually, liver. Such congestion may well be the leading cause of cancer and other degenerative diseases. It often comes back to the liver. When toxins are not purged from the system quickly enough, they get reabsorbed through the intestinal wall back into the bloodstream. From here they are carried back to the liver, which filtered from the bloodstream for their removal in the first place.

The 80/20 diet, built on foods from the plant kingdom, is a smorgasbord of fiber. Your colon and liver will thank you. Your whole body—even your stubborn taste buds—will eventually thank you.

NEED MEAL IDEAS?

If I've convinced you of how important raw foods are to your health, you may wish to order from Health*Quarters* a copy of a cookbook I put together called *Raw, Raw, Raw.* It presents an 80/20 strategy:

- Raw fruits and fruit juices for breakfast
- Raw veggies and salads for lunch
- Something raw and something cooked for dinner

Follow this schedule, and you're pretty well assured of eating at least 80 percent of your daily intake of food in its raw form. You can be flexible, adding more cooked if you wish. However, if you're fighting cancer, let me encourage you to eat as much as possible raw—and if at all possible, organically grown.

CAN'T DIGEST RAW FOODS?

If you have trouble digesting raw produce, it's not the food that needs to change but your digestion. Most Americans over the age of 30 don't make enough hydrochloric acid in their stomachs to properly digest foods. Gas, bloating, indigestion, mucus, undigested food in a bowel movement, and so on, are signs. If you suspect that like 9 out of 10 adult Americans you are underacid, let me suggest that you do the following:

- Remove all caffeine and sugar from your diet (these destroy B vitamins and use up precious minerals).

- Add B-vitamins and multiminerals to your supplement program (your stomach uses these to help make hydrochloric acid).

- Take four capsules per meal of a product called Food Enzymes (for at least a month while your body is rebuilding its ability to make sufficient hydrochloric acid; be sure to take these after there is food already in your stomach).

ENZYMES

The following items mentioned in this chapter are all available from Health*Quarters* Ministries. You may be able to find all but the cookbook in health food stores as well.

- *Raw, Raw, Raw* (80/20 cookbook)

- B-vitamins (of highest quality and potency)

- Super Supplemental (without iron)

- Food Enzymes (a blend of hydrochloric acid, bile salt, bromelain, lipase, mycozyme, pancreatin, papain, and pepsin)

20

HORMONE BALANCING WITH NATURAL PROGESTERONE

ONE OF THE MOST IMPORTANT strategies in any effective cancer battle plan is the balancing of hormones. Hormones are chemical messengers sent out from certain glands to tell various parts of the body what to do. When hormones become unbalanced—too much of one, not enough of another—the system goes haywire.

Supplementing with natural progesterone cream (the kind derived from certain fats found in Mexican wild yams, not the synthetic forms like Provera and other "progestins") is important. After reading the following, you may conclude that it is absolutely fundamental.

Here are some facts to consider.

IN WOMEN

Fact: The two primary hormones produced are estrogen and progesterone. A healthy balance in the female body is 10 progesterone to 1 estrogen.

Fact: Progesterone production begins to decrease about age 35, tailing off to nearly zero approaching menopause. At the same time, estrogen production, although decreasing as well, remains much greater than progesterone.

Fact: Estrogen dominance (unbalanced estrogen) is a primary cause in almost all female health problems, including: fibrocystic breast disease, PMS, mood swings, decreased libido, thyroid dysfunction, water retention, excessive bleeding, endometriosis, fibroids, infertility, ovarian cysts, increased fat storage, tissue damage, bruising and pigment discoloration on the face, aging of the skin, pituitary gland damage, and poor liver function.

Fact: Estrogen dominance is also the only known cause of uterine cancer. In the mid-1970s it was recognized by medical science that giving women estrogen replacement therapy (ERT) led to an increase in the incidence of uterine cancer.[1] Yet it was thought that estrogen needed to be given to help combat osteoporosis. (Excess estrogen in the female body is also a leading cause of breast and ovarian cancers.)

Fact: New studies now show that estrogen does little more than slow bone loss, while progesterone actually helps to build new bone. John R. Lee, M.D., the "guru" of hormone replacement therapy, takes all his patients off estrogen and puts them on a program of progesterone along with diet changes and supplements. He claims virtually 100 percent success in building bone mass.[2]

Fact: The same studies are also showing conclusive evidence that estrogen replacement therapy does indeed actually promote and feed cancer, while progesteron inhibits it.[3]

Conclusion: It's a "no brainer." Add natural progesterone to your cancer battle plan. "It would be wise to phase off the estrogen as soon as possible (if you're currently on it) and replace it with natural progesterone," says Dr. Joseph Mercola. "If hot flashes are a problem, a phytoestrogen like black cohosh is generally effective."[4]

Note: Besides being the result of a naturally occurring decrease in progesterone, estrogen dominance is compounded by: (1) poor blood and lymph circulation and sluggish elimination, which hinders the liver, kidney, and colon from being able to process and eliminate excess estrogen; (2) consumption of animal products that stimulate the body's natural estrogen production—a "double whammy," since it's become standard practice to feed estrogens to livestock to fatten them quickly for market; and (3) consumption of foods that have been sprayed with pesticides and herbicides, since studies show that they mimic estrogen in the body.

Breast cancer cells do not multiply when women are on progesterone.

JOSEPH M. MERCOLA, D.O.

IN MEN

Fact: The primary hormone produced is testosterone. Men also produce about half as much progesterone as women, and a little estrogen.

Fact: Recent studies show that testosterone does not cause prostate cancer (as has been commonly thought in some circles) but actually prevents estrogen from doing so by destroying the prostate cancer cells it stimulates. Estrogen stimulates both enlargement of, and cancer cell development in, the prostate gland.[5]

Fact: It's a man's progesterone that keeps his testosterone strong. When progesterone production begins to decrease at around age 45, a naturally occurring enzyme, 5-alpha reductase, turns strong testosterone into "whimpy" testosterone, useless at destroying prostate cancer cells that estrogen stimulates. In other words, men need good supplies of progesterone to keep their testosterone healthy in order to balance the effects of their estrogen.[6]

Fact: Studies show that progesterone appears to work better at inhibiting the testosterone-converting impact of 5-alpha reductase than do the popularly used Proscar (pharmaceutical) or saw palmetto (an herbal product).[7]

Conclusion: It's another "no brainer"! Add natural progesterone to your cancer battle plan.

WHAT KIND OF PROGESTERONE IS BEST?

Progesterone is best utilized by the body transdermally, when applied to the skin in cream form. The hormone is absorbed directly into the bloodstream, bypassing any breakdown that might occur in the digestive system or liver. Creams also deliver their hormone content in a more gradual, steady fashion than capsules or oils taken orally.

Although progesterone cream is made from Mexican wild yam extract, Mexican wild yam extract itself is not yet progesterone. Don't be fooled. The word "progesterone" must be listed as an ingredient in whatever product you purchase. The body cannot metabolize wild yam extract into usable progesterone. This must be done in a lab setting before it is made into the cream.

There are many progesterone creams on the market. You want one that contains at least 450 milligrams of natural progesterone per ounce and doesn't come with toxic cosmetic ingredients. John Lee, M.D., recommends Pro-Gest, the brand we carry and heartily endorse at HealthQuarters Ministries. We've received lots of good feedback.

How much to use? Read the instructions that come with the product. Normally males use ¼ teaspoon twice a day. Females need about twice as much, or ½ teaspoon twice a day. Men can take it on an ongoing basis. Nonmenopausal women need time off each month in relationship to their menstrual cycle. Dr. Mercola suggests using it only days 12 to 26.

More is not better when it comes to progesterone. Too much can be counterproductive.

Pro-Gest brand progesterone cream and the books can all be ordered from HealthQuarters Ministries. They may also be available at your local health food store.

FURTHER READING

All four of these books are extraordinarily helpful for developing a thorough understanding of the female body and its unique health needs. I have all four in my personal library and would like to encourage you to do the same, whether you're female or male. They are available through Health-Quarters Ministries.

Alternative Medicine Guide to Women's Health 1, by Burton Goldberg and the editors of *Alternative Medicine* (Tiburon, CA: Future Medicine, 1998).

Alternative Medicine Guide to Women's Health 2, by Burton Goldberg and the editors of *Alternative Medicine* (Tiburon, CA: Future Medicine, 1998).

What Your Doctor May Not Tell You about Menopause, by John R. Lee (New York: Warner Books), 1996.

What Your Doctor May Not Tell You about Premenopause, by John R. Lee (New York: Warner Books), 1996.

21

EXERCISE, SUNSHINE, SLEEP

THE HUMAN BODY is a "machine" that requires use to get and remain strong. If you're not getting stronger, you're getting weaker. A day without exercise is a day in decline. Daily exercise is a fundamental part of maintaining the body in good health for the long haul. It is also an important part of any ef-fective cancer battle plan. Exercise

- drains the lymph system, part of the garbage disposal system in the body; a sluggish lymph system sets the stage for the development of disease

- stimulates the removal of toxic wastes through the colon, skin, and lungs; cancer thrives in a toxic environment

- generates a sense of well-being by stimulating the release of endor-phins from the pituitary gland that act as a type of natural morphine; a positive attitude aids the immune system

- stimulates natural killer (NK) cell activity

- oxygenates the cells and tissues; cancer can't survive in an oxygenated environment

Walk!

ANDREW WEIL, M.D.,
Spontaneous Healing

TWO KEY FORMS

For an individual who is fighting cancer, I suggest two forms of exercise in order to reap the rewards just listed:

- Rebounding

    (see chapter 16)

- Walking

    Comfortable shoes are a must.

    Start at 30 minutes a day, three days a week.

    Work toward 60 minutes a day, six to seven days a week.

    Swing your arms.

    Keep a steady pace. Be brisk, but not so fast that you get "winded."

SUNSHINE

Used properly, the sun is a significant partner in one's quest for health and healing. The benefits of sunshine are numerous. Sunshine

- converts ergosterol found just below the skin into vitamin D, which helps the body absorb and retain calcium

- promotes the use of oxygen in our tissues

- lowers blood sugar levels in the bloodstream

- stimulates the thyroid gland, thus increasing metabolism

- stimulates white blood cells, thus increasing the power and potential of the immune system

- has a positive effect on hormone balance

- stimulates the production of neurotransmitters in the brain that keep mood elevated

- Inhibits the development of breast and colon cancer

Keys to Effective Sun Use

- Sunbathe, don't sunburn. It is suggested we get at least 30 minutes of sunshine every day on as much of our body as possible. The best hours for such "bathing" tend to be before 10 a.m. and after 3 p.m., when the sun's rays are less intense.

Combining your "sun time" with a morning or afternoon walk is a great idea. Even during the winter in cold climates, get out and get some sun on your skin whenever possible.

- When in the sun for extended periods, protect your skin with clothing and/or sunscreen. You should be able to find a sunscreen product at your local health food store that does not contain toxic chemicals. Look for one with protective herbs and nutrients such as vitamins A, C, and E, lycopene, selenium, zinc, witch hazel, aloe, milk thistle, calendula, and plantain. Make sure other ingredients are nontoxic by checking them against listings in books like *A Consumer's Dictionary of Cosmetic Ingredients,* by Ruth Winter, M.S.

- Eliminate or at least cut way back on animal fats in your diet. It's the animal fats in the standard American diet (S.A.D.) that wound skin, making it more apt to burn and eventually develop skin cancer.

- Do include essential fatty acids in your diet. Flaxseed oil is the highest plant source of Omega-3 and is a good source of Omega-6 fatty acids. Together they help to build strong cells and are important for overall skin health. Take 1 or 2 tablespoons straight, or mix with things like oatmeal or smoothies.

- Eat lots of carrots; drink lots of carrot juice. Veggies, especially carrots, contain lots of carotenes. These raise the threshold at which your skin will burn.

- Take antioxidant supplements. Antioxidant nutrients like vitamins A, C, E, selenium, zinc, pine bark and grape seed extracts, and many more protect your skin from free radical damage.

- Drink lots of water. Adequate water consumption ensures that your skin cells stay hydrated. Dehydrated skin cells are more susceptible to sunburn and aging.

SLEEP

Learning how to effectively rest your body is a fundamental part of being a good caretaker of your long-term health. In chapter 7, I discussed poor sleep habits as part of a toxic lifestyle. In fact, 70 percent of the healing and restoration of your body from the rigors of daily life and/or the impact of illnesses and disease processes takes place while you're asleep.

TRY THESE TO GET YOUR Z'S

Here's my list of seven things to try in an effort to help rest your body more efficiently and effectively.

1. Deal with issues of heart and head before you hit the bed. Studies done in sleep labs show evidence that up to 50 percent of all sleep problems are caused by psychological factors. Let me suggest two things to do every night before bed:

- *Get it out of your mind.* Make a "do list" for the next day before going to bed. Write it all down and forget it. Next to my computer on my desk at home I have posted a list of things I make it my aim to accomplish every day. Get it out of your mind and onto paper.

- *Get it off your chest.* Before crawling under the covers, spend a moment or two reviewing the day. There's nothing like a clear conscience to help induce peaceful sleep. Stress keeps the brain turned on, tuned in, and ready for battle. The Bible talks about not letting the sun go down on your anger.

2. Develop a habit of regular exercise. Exercise has been shown to help improve the quality of sleep. It triggers certain biochemical changes in the body that help to enable restful sleep. Morning exercise is best, and early evening is good, too.

3. Avoid dietary sleep-robbers. Stimulants like sugar, alcohol, and caffeine (coffee, tea, chocolate, soft drinks, cocoa), included in your daily diet at all, should be consumed no later than about five hours before bedtime.

4. Prepare the bedroom. The environment in your bedroom contributes to the quality of sleep you'll experience. Here are a few tips:

- *Air temperature.* It's a fact that most folks sleep better in a cool environment. I sleep with my window cracked just a bit, even during Colorado winters, to get cool and fresh air circulating in my bedroom. I also pile my bed high with blankets.

- *Air quality.* Keep that window cracked in order to bring in fresh air. Or you might also want to consider an air purification system (see chapter 22) for your bedroom, especially if you're in a newer home.

Summary

1. Deal with issues of the heart and head before you hit the bed.
   - Get it out of your mind (do list)
   - Get it off your chest (get right with God, and spouse)
2. Develop a habit of regular exercise. "If you don't rev up during the day, you'll have a harder time revving down during the night."
3. Avoid dietary sleep-robbers. Sugar, alcohol, caffeine (if any, none after about 5 p.m.)
4. Prepare the bedroom.
   - Air temperature
   - Air quality
   - Sound
   - Light
5. Develop a rhythm. Go to bed and get up at the same time every day.

(continued on next page)

If you have recently put down new carpet in the bedroom or sleep above a garage with parked cars, there will be considerable outgassing of toxic gases into the breathing air.

- *Sound.* This is a subjective area. Some folks sleep with a small fan running nearby that muffles other noises in the house and provides a soothing rhythm. Other folks can't go to sleep if there's any noise whatsoever. Discover what's best for you. Perhaps an Alpine Air Purification system will be just the thing, providing both fan noise and purification.

- *Light.* Melatonin, a hormone produced by the pineal gland (a small gland in the brain), controls our sleep cycles and helps us to rest soundly. When it begins to get dark, the pineal gland begins to release melatonin to help us sleep. When it begins to get light, melatonin release is stopped in order to prepare for alertness.

   The darker your bedroom, the more likely you are to enjoy a good night's sleep because of the melatonin released by the pineal gland in the presence of full darkness. A night light in the room or light from the moon streaming through the curtains or a neighbor's porchlight can all impact the amount of melatonin released from the pineal gland.

5. Develop a rhythm. Life revolves around day and night, light and dark.

   The human body has a daily rhythm of its own, referred to as the circadian rhythm. From about 4 a.m. to noon is a cycle referred to as Elimination. The primary working of the body during this time frame is the flushing out of body wastes and food debris from what was eaten the day before. Noon to 8 p.m. is titled Appropriation, for that's when the body wants most to be fed and to do its work of digestion. And finally, the cycle from about 8 p.m. to 4 a.m. is called Assimilation. This is the time when the body works its best and hardest to absorb and use nutrients to build and repair itself.

   It would seem best to practice getting to be early and get up early—in tune with the 8 p.m.–to–4 a.m. cycle. With the advent of electricity, we've actually lost touch with the natural rhythms of our own system. Scientists who study sleep tell us that the body values the hours of sleep before midnight as twice as important as those after midnight. If you got to bed by 10 p.m., then by midnight on your body's clock you've already had four hours of sleep. If you then got up at 4 a.m., you will have logged the equivalent of eight hours—again based on the fact that the body puts double value on premidnight hours.

It matters not only when you go to bed, but that you do so at the same time every night. Our bodies are governed by, and thus are most comfortable when operating on, a repeated schedule—a rhythm. This serves to enhance the ebb and flow of your energies. It is good to begin doing your bedtime routine—brushing your teeth, flossing, reading a book, or whatever—each night about 30 minutes before hitting the sheets, as it signals your body and mind to begin to wind down.

What if you have a job where you work hours that violate these daily cycles—the graveyard shift in some factory or the third shift in a hospital? Or, even worse, what if you work varying shifts? You're probably going to pay some price in your health. Taking supplemental melatonin may be helpful (more about that follows).

6. Take an essential oils soak (see chapter 15, "Soaks and Saunas").

7. Take a sleep aid. When people don't get the sleep their bodies require, their health and healing potential suffer. The following nondrug sleep aids are available from your local health food store, and from Health*Quarters*.

- *Melatonin* (tells the brain to sleep). Melatonin controls our sleep cycles and helps us to rest soundly. When it begins to get dark, the pineal gland begins to release melatonin to help us sleep. When it begins to get light, melatonin release is stopped in order to prepare for alertness. Studies show that, as we age, we tend to produce less and less of this important hormone, and the result is bouts of sleeplessness.

  Night shift workers and people who experience jet lag while they travel have discovered that melatonin helps resolve their sleep problems. Not only is melatonin important for sleep production, but evidence is mounting that it serves many additional purposes in the body.

  A daily supplement of this hormone could help humans stay younger and healthier as they age. Melatonin seems to direct the process of aging. When the melatonin-producing pineal glands of young mice were transplanted into old mice, the old mice became

Summary

(continued from previous page)

6. Take an essential oils soak (see chapter 15, "Soaks and Saunas").
7. Try a sleep aid.
   - Melatonin (tells the brain to sleep)
   - GABA (quiets the brain's response to stress)
   - Magnesium malate (relaxes the muscles and nervous system)

stronger and their hair grew thicker. When the pineal glands of old mice were transplanted into young mice, they started to age rapidly, lost hair, got cataracts in their eyes, and hobbled around. This study, along with others, provides growing evidence of melatonin combating the effects of aging.

In other mice studies, melatonin also appears to keep the thymus gland and the immune system strong, as well as to function in the system as an antioxidant, protecting it from the ravages of free radicals. Studies done on humans to this point show that melatonin may reduce breast tumors and gastric cancers.

Research suggests that melatonin supplements are not addictive and do replenish depleted stores of this hormone in the system. It is advisable, however, to use melatonin on an "as needed" basis, not daily. You want your body to be able to produce more melatonin by itself. That said, you will be glad you've got a supply of Melatonin Extra on hand the next time you're faced with a sleepless night.

- *Gamma-aminobutyric acid (GABA)* (dampens the brain's response to stress). GABA is an amino acid essential for proper brain function. GABA's role in the brain is to decrease neuron activity and inhibit nerve cells from overfiring. Together with a couple of key nutrients from the vitamin B family, niacinamide and inositol, it prevents anxiety and stress messages from reaching and stimulating the motor centers of the brain. GABA can be taken to calm the body in much the same way as Valium or Librium, and other tranquilizers, but without fear of addiction.

  I've taken GABA myself on the recommendation of a medical doctor friend and have found it to be a helpful sleep aid.

- *Magnesium malate* (relaxes the muscles and nervous system). Have you ever awakened from sleep with a "charlie horse"? Whenever you experience muscle cramping of any kind, think magnesium. This nutrient is known as the muscle relaxant mineral. Generally speaking, most Americans are low in it. Emotional stress, loud noise, sugar, alcohol, and caffeine rob the body of magnesium stores. And if you are fighting cancer, it's generally true that your magnesium stores have been even more depleted.

22

AIR AND WATER PURIFICATION STRATEGIES

AIR IS THE SINGLE MOST IMPORTANT nutrient for human health. Water is second. It's important that your intake of both is as clean as possible.

AIR

In chapter 6, I discussed the pollution problems found in much indoor air. The EPA is concerned with three categories of these pollutants:

1. Particulates like bacteria, viruses, fungi, dander, pollens, and other microbes

2. Gases like formaldehyde emitted from manmade materials

3. Radon, a toxic gas generated by the breakdown of rock and soil

In chapter 9, I discussed the value of deep breathing in an effort to help detoxify the body. Obviously, clean air is essential.

FOUR STRATEGIES FOR CLEANING UP INDOOR AIR

1. *Eliminate.* You need to remove from your breathing space anything that has the potential to outgas toxic gases or throw off particulates.

- *Ban smoking.* Tobacco smoke releases over four thousand toxic gases into the air, including carbon monoxide and formaldehyde. Smoking turns an indoor air environment into a literal gas chamber.

- *Switch to nontoxic household cleaning products.* Read the labels, and you will find that some scouring powders contain chlorine. You'll do your health a big favor by going with the nonchlorinated kind. Plain old baking soda makes a wonderful, nontoxic scouring agent.

  Another nontoxic choice would be to use vinegar and water to clean windows rather than an ammonia-based spray; ¼ cup of white vinegar and 1 teaspoon of baking soda mixed in a gallon of water is a good all-purpose cleaner.

- *Consider getting rid of your carpet.* Carpet can be one of the most toxic things in your home or office. New carpet outgasses as many as 60 toxic chemicals—some up to 15 years. Many of these act like estrogens in the body.

  Old carpets harbor dust, dust mites, and a host of microbes like disease-causing viruses and bacteria. As carpet breaks down, fibers escape into the air, carrying those microbes with them. Not only is the carpet itself potentially bad news, but the pad on which it lies can be even more toxic. If you've got hardwood floors beneath your carpet, let them show.

- *Cook your house.* Close the windows, turn up the heat, and leave for several days. Before you come back to stay, air out the place for several hours. Some authorities suggest this as a method for accelerating the outgassing of products, especially in a new home.

2. *Ventilate.*

- *Adopt an open-window policy.* This is particularly important in your bedroom. Keep a window cracked open year round. Seventy percent of our body's healing and restoration takes place while we sleep. Fresh air is important to this process. (Note: if your bedroom is above your garage, don't park your car in there. Outgassing fumes will penetrate the air space.)

- *Check for radon.* Radon is a radioactive gas originating primarily from the breakdown of uranium in rock and soil. You can't smell, see, or taste it. It tends to seep into a house through cracks in the foundation or unfinished floors in crawl spaces. It can also come into a home by way of tap water, evaporating into the air space.

  The Surgeon General has labeled radon the second leading cause of lung cancer.

  To have your home checked, look under "Radon" in your yellow pages. You can purchase do-it-yourself test kits from many hardware and even grocery stores. Just follow the instructions. If you house is found to have a problem, there are special contractors listed in the same area of the phone book who design solutions for venting the radon from your home.

3. *Decorate.* Dr. Bill Wolverton, a former NASA scientist, talks in his book *How to Grow Fresh Air* about how, as plans for a manned moon base were developed, he and fellow scientists studied the issue of how to both generate and clean the moon base air supply. They ran tests during various space missions and discovered that those who traveled inside spacecraft were exposed to more than three hundred different toxic gases. Chief among these was formaldehyde.

In 1980, they discovered that regular houseplants could effectively and efficiently clean indoor air of a host of toxic gases, including the ubiquitous formaldehyde. The subtitle of Wolverton's book is *50 Houseplants That Purify Your Home or Office.* Each plant is pictured with a rating of its air-purifying effectiveness and instructions as to how to grow it.

I love his book! I think you will too.

4. *Purificate.* Within this particular strategy, there are at least two techniques:

- Diffusing essential oils into the air (see chapter 23, "Aromatherapy")
- Using an air purification system

At Health*Quarters* Ministries we make available the Alpine air purification system. We use one to clean our own office air. The Alpine is not a filter, though. Filters are only partially effective in cleaning up indoor air. They can only clean the air that happens to flow through them, and even then can only remove particulates. They have no impact on gases.

The Alpine air purification system purifies indoor air in a way similar to the way a thunderstorm purifies outdoor air.

When lightning hits oxygen in the atmosphere, an activated form of oxygen called ozone is created. This activated oxygen serves to break down and oxidize gaseous pollutants in the air. The same bolt of lightning also creates what are called negative ions. These attract toxic particles floating in the air, bringing them to the ground.

You might say that ozone and negative ions are the dynamic duo that God uses to clean the world's atmosphere. I enjoy a walk outside just after a thunderstorm. The air is clean and fresh.

In a similar fashion, the Alpine uses existing air and an electrical charge to create ozone and negative ions. Toxic gases are neutralized. Particulates like mold, mildew, fungi, bacteria, and viruses are bound and dropped out of the breathing air.

The Alpine comes in several different models. The biggest one is the XL-15. The size of a four-slice toaster, it cleans the air space in up to 2,500 square feet. There are smaller units for smaller areas, even one that will plug into the cigarette lighter of a vehicle.

Note: There are some who warn about the wounding impact of too much ozone on the lungs. Control knobs allow for variation of the amount of ozone emitted. A low level is good when people are in the air space being cleaned. Turning up the ozone now and then when the office closes or no one will be in the home is a great way to thoroughly wash the indoor air. Simply ventilate before people return for extended use.

How to Grow Fresh Air by Dr. Bill Wolverton may be available in your local book or health food store. You also may be able to find an Alpine dealer in your yellow pages. Both the book and the purifier are also available from Health*Quarters.*

WATER

Second only to air in its importance to your health is water. In chapter 10, I discussed the importance of keeping your body well hydrated with water in the effort to "unload" the body of toxins. It's important that your drinking water be purified. If you're in the midst of a cancer battle plan, do not drink tap water! It has become "chemical soup" and is stressful on a compromised system that has allowed cancer cells to thrive. Each glass will further burden an overwhelmed liver that is in charge of cleaning toxic poisons from the bloodstream. Drinking from the tap is like shooting yourself in the proverbial foot.

THREE FORMS OF WATER PURIFICATION

Carbon filtration will not accomplish all that needs to be done, as illustrated in the following table. It is true that a carbon filter on a shower head will help to keep you from breathing chlorine into your lungs during a shower; however, this is not sufficient purification for drinking water.

Although a distiller may make the most absolutely pure water, I'm a fan of reverse osmosis (RO) filtering systems. They do a comparable job, don't need a power source, and don't heat up the house. Not only that, but RO water tastes better to me than distilled. Nevertheless, either would be a good choice to have in your home.

Removal Summary*	Carbon Filters	RO Systems	Distillers
Tastes/odors	Yes	Yes	Yes
Organic chemicals: fertilizers, pesticides, herbicides, paints, fuels, cleansing agents, human and animal wastes, etc.	Yes	Yes	Yes
Additives: chlorine, fluoride	Just chlorine	Yes	Yes
Inorganic minerals/ metals: calcium, magnesium, iron, manganese, aluminum, arsenic, asbestos, barium, cadmium, chromium, copper, fluoride, lead, mercury, nitrate, nitrite, selenium, silver	No	Yes	Yes
Radioactive substances: manmade radioactive minerals, radon gas	Just radon	Yes	Yes
Microorganisms: bacteria, viruses, parasites	No	All in theory, most in practice	Yes

*The information in this table is from Colin Ingram's exhaustive work *The Drinking Water Book* (Berkeley, CA: Ten Speed Press, 1991).

There are many sources for RO water filtering systems and distillers. A check of your yellow pages will no doubt turn up several. If you wish to bypass such a purchase, you may be able to have RO or distilled water delivered to your home from a company specializing in such a service.

I have an under-the-sink RO system for my own kitchen. Two models of a high-quality, low-cost RO system are available from Health*Quarters*— both four-filter and five-filter machines.

23

ESSENTIAL OILS AND AROMATHERAPY

AROMATHERAPY IS THE TERM used to describe the use of "essential oils" (oils derived from various plant sources) to benefit the human body in various ways. Although the term would lead one to think that the exclusive way in which these oils are used is to diffuse (vaporize) them as aromatic scents into breathing space, they are perhaps even more effective when applied directly to the skin.

HOW ESSENTIAL OILS WORK

Use of essential oils can do at least three things for the human body: recharge its electrical frequency; deliver nutrients to cells; and change brain/body chemistry.

Recharging the Body's Electrical Frequency
Everything that "is" puts off a measurable electrical frequency. That's because everything that "is" is made of atoms, which have electrons whizzing about them, creating an electromagnetic field. Your body, being made of atoms, puts off its own frequency. One might say that you're a "humming" being—a "bioelectrical" battery. A healthy body typically has a frequency

"Clinical research shows," writes Gary Young, N.D., "that essential oils have the highest frequency of any natural substance known to man, creating an environment in which disease, bacteria, virus, fungus, etc., cannot live. I believe that the chemistry and frequencies of essential oils have the ability to help man maintain the optimal frequency to the extent that disease cannot exist."

ranging from 62 to 78 Hertz (Hz). In disease the body's electrical frequency has dropped to 58 Hz.[1]

What can be done to help "power up" and protect a person's electrical frequency? Many point toward the use of essential oils as a very important tool.

Research studies have discovered the following frequencies:[2]

Processed/canned food	0 Hz (electrically dead)
Fresh produce	up to 15 Hz
Dry herbs	12–22 Hz
Fresh herbs	20–27 Hz
Essential oils	start at 52 Hz and go up to 320 Hz

The conclusion many draw from these studies is that the use of essential oils, either inhaled or applied to the skin, can help to revive and strengthen the electrical frequency of the body's cells.

Delivering Nutrients to Cells

Essential oils are to plants what blood is to the human body. They contain oxygen (a nutrient transporter) and an array of nutrients that give life to the plant. When these oils are diffused into the air, tiny molecules containing the oxygen and plant nutrients are released. What our noses perceive as an "odor" is actually an "airborne meal." When these vapors are inhaled, the oxygen and nutrient–rich molecules are diffused through our lungs into our bloodstream. The oxygen serves to carry the plant-derived nutrients via our blood to every cell in our bodies.

A more direct, and some say more effective, way to get essential oils into the body is to apply them in diluted form directly to the skin ("topically"). In this way they are absorbed quickly and efficiently into the bloodstream. The feet are often the site of choice when applying essential oils, since the biggest skin pores are located there. The nutrients in the oil are quickly absorbed and transported throughout the body, affecting every cell, including the hair, within 20 minutes.[3]

Changing Brain Chemistry

Besides being electrically and nutritionally therapeutic in their impact on the body, essential oils are also neurologically therapeutic. They have a "mind-altering" impact on the brain via its limbic system (the neurological processing center that, among other things, translates smell into emotion).

When a specific smell stimulates the limbic system of the brain through its sensory connection with the nasal passages, the chemistry of the brain is altered and certain emotions are generated. With specific emotions come related hormonal messengers sent forth by the brain to tell the various other body parts how to respond. Thus, in a fascinating domino effect, odors impact the workings of the whole body.

As an example of how "essential oil" vapors affect brain chemistry, I have a friend who suffers from seasonal affective disorder (S.A.D.)—depression caused by lack of sunlight. If skies are cloudy and she goes for too many days without sunshine, the "blues" overwhelm her. And since every cell in the body is impacted by emotions generated by the brain, immune power fades out as depression sets in. Sickness is not far behind.

However, diffusing a little essential oil of lemon or orange now and then into her breathing space changes everything. Even though the sun may not be shining, her smile is. The depression lifts. Immune power fires back up. And all is right with the world once again.

This is just one of many examples of how essential oils affect the brain and the rest of the body. Lest you conclude that vapors are little more than a placebo, bringing with them certain expectations of changed mood, studies done on animals (who carry with them no expectations) show the same changes in behavior that humans experience when exposed to various vapors.

Properties of Some Common Scents

Black cumin—supports the immune system

Cinnamon bark—fights viruses and infectious diseases

Cistus—supports and strengthens immune power

Clove—anti-infectious, antibacterial, antiviral, antifungal, antiparasitic, antiseptic

Cypress—helps decongest the lymph system

Davana—helps stimulate the glandular system

Dill—helps support the pancreas

Eucalyptus—anti-infectious, antibacterial, antiviral

Frankincense—fights tumors, stimulates the immune system

Galbanum—strengthens the body overall

Lemon—promotes white blood cell formation, increases lymphatic function

Melaluca—anti-infectious, antibacterial, antifungal, antiviral, antiparasitic, stimulates the immune system

Mountain savory—stimulates the immune system

Myrrh—supports the immune system, decongests the prostate gland

Myrtle—helps the immune system, normalizes hormonal imbalances

Neroli—antibacterial, antiviral, antiparasitic, anti-infectious

Oregano—antiviral, antibacterial, antifungal, antiparasitic

Rose—balances whole body, enhances frequency of every cell

Rosemary—strengthens immune system, helps glandular system

Sandalwood—increases oxygen to pituitary and pineal glands

Spearmint—helps open/release emotional blocks, bring balance

Spruce—helps the glandular system, helps open/release emotional blocks

Thyme—supports the immune system; antimicrobial, antifungal, antibacterial, antiviral; helps overcome fatigue and weakness

Wild tansy—supports the immune system

These are but a few of the hundreds of essential oils on the market today, with each having many more benefits than listed here. As a naturopath and nutritionist I enjoy using essential oils to help folks protect and/or win back their health. Essential oils ought to be in your cancer-fighting toolbox.

Essential oils and products containing them are available in stores across the nation. Those manufactured by the network-marketing company Young Living are regarded by most in this field as superior in quality. Check your yellow pages for a Young Living Essential Oils distributor near you, or you may obtain a catalog and order directly from the company. To do so, you must give a sponsor's member number when you call (1-800-763-9963). If you wish, you may use Health*Quarters* Ministries as your sponsoring agent (member # 217162). You'll hear automated instructions. At their conclusion press 3 on your touch tone phone to talk to a live operator. You'll be given your own member number to use from then on whenever you order.

24

WATER AND
HYDROTHERAPY

HAVE YOU HEARD about those hearty Norwegian folk who like to sit in shacks working up a sweat, then run out and jump through a hole cut in a frozen lake? Crazy? Such a practice can do wonders for one's health. The variation in temperature accomplishes the following:

- Contracts and dilates the blood vessels

- Multiplies oxygen supply in the blood

- Improves circulation and delivery of nutrients to vital areas

- Activates organ function

- Hastens removal of toxins

- Increases the number of white blood cells in circulation

- Stimulates the glandular system (pituitary, pineal, thyroid, thymus, pancreas, and adrenals)

- Reduces congestion

- Alleviates inflammation

What those folks are practicing is a form of hydrotherapy, the use of water (in this case, COLD water) and/or temperature variation to stimulate the body's own healing powers.

There are many other forms of hydrotherapy, including, for example, various kinds of soaks and saunas to help remove toxins through the skin (which I discussed in chapter 15) and the use of hot and/or cold showers to enhance healing.

USING YOUR SHOWER TO STRENGTHEN YOUR HEALING POWER

If you've got a shower in your home, you have access to a wonderful, cheap, easily used tool for strengthening your immune system to protect you against cancer cells, bacterial and viral infections, parasites, and so on.

All the benefits those Nordic types gain from heating up their bodies and plunging them into frozen lakes can be yours without leaving the comfort of your home. Here's how.

1. Stand in a shower for three minutes, as hot as you can stand it without scalding your skin.

2. For 30 seconds, turn the water as cold as you can stand it without having a heart attack. (Gasping? Gasping is good! Helps to oxygenate the body.)

3. Do this variation sequence three times, ending with cold.

4. Towel off briskly.

5. Do this on a regular basis.

All the listed benefits will be yours.

A WORD OR TWO ABOUT HYPERTHERMIA

Hyperthermia is a form of hydrotherapy performed under the care of a qualified doctor. Fever is intentionally induced (by raising the overall body temperature) in a body that is having a hard time generating such a response on its own to disease-causing agents. Contrary to popular belief, fevers are not something to suppress but a natural response by the body to help destroy invading pathogens.

I'm amazed at how often people with cancer will tell me they can't believe they have the disease, for they haven't been sick in years. The truth is, their immune systems haven't been strong enough to mount an offensive against an invading pathogen. Colds, flu, and fevers are signs of a body hard at work. To have one or two minor colds a year is not unusual for a healthy person.

FURTHER READING

Hydrotherapy, by Clarence Dail and Charles Thomas (Brushton, NY: TEACH
   Services, 1995).

25

MAGNET THERAPY

MAGNETS HAVE ATTRACTED attention in the field of health for centuries. Recent years have seen a re-emergence of their popularity. It is estimated that in 1997 alone, Americans bought therapeutic magnets to the tune of $500 million.[1]

Are they useful in a cancer battle plan?

"I have seen dramatic results when the north magnetic pole is applied to a cancer or an area of inflammation," says Dr. Michael Schachter, M.D.[2] He points out that the north, or negative, pole tends to inhibit inflammation and cancer growth, while the south stimulates both.

HOW DO MAGNETS WORK?

Researchers have discovered the following facts about the impact of fixed magnetic energy upon the human body.[3]

North and south magnetic poles act in opposite ways.

North (the negative magnetic energy pole):

- Attracts oxygen
- Arrests bacteria

- Stops growths

- Controls inflammatory conditions (swelling)

- Reduces congestion

- Inhibits pain

- Contracts tissues

- Constricts blood vessels

- Slows overactive organs

- Increases alkalinity

- Reduces acidity

- Controls bleeding/coagulation of blood

- Dissolves buildup of fatty deposits

- Reverses effects of electromagnetic pollution

    South (the positive magnetic pole):

- Stimulates growth of bacteria

- Stimulates organ function

- Causes acidity

- Expands, enlarges, softens, and relaxes tissues

- Dilates blood vessels

Obviously, the north pole of a magnet is the one most often applied in therapy. South is rarely, if ever, used. It's also important to point out that magnets heal nothing but serve to stimulate and facilitate the body's healing processes—a theme common to all the "tools" mentioned in this book.

WHAT CONDITIONS DO THEY HELP?

In the November 1997 issue of *Archives of Physical Medicine and Rehabilitation,* research results were published that captured considerable attention. A double-blind, placebo-controlled study documented that magnet therapy gave quick relief to folks suffering from post-polio pain. Studies over the years have shown the use of permanent magnets to be of benefit to the following conditions: arthritis, whiplash, backaches, head injuries, headaches, diabetes, kidney infections, kidney stones, cancer, bladder problems, dental surgeries, menstrual pain, knee inflammation, carpal tunnel syndrome, infections, hormonal imbalances, fatigue, eczema and other skin rashes,

sciatica, sinusitis, toothache, bone and skin grafts, vertigo and motion sickness, insomnia, glaucoma, sexual problems . . . and more.

HOW DO YOU USE THEM?

Therapeutic magnets are marked as to which side is north. They can be
purchased as singles or sewn into the lining of various-sized wraps, pillow
inserts, mattress pads, shoe insoles, and so on. The north (negative) magnetic field is always positioned to face the body.

I often wear a magnetic wrap around my waist to minister to an aching
lower back, and another around my sometimes sore left knee. My next purchase? A magnetic mattress pad. I'm looking forward to keeping my entire
body exposed to negative magnetic field for eight hours a night.

Magnetic therapy is extremely safe, user friendly, and a "no-brainer."

Many retail department stores now carry a variety of therapeutic magnet
products, as do health food stores. You may also want to give Health*Quarters* a call. We will be able to meet your need or point you in an appropriate
direction.

FURTHER READING

Biomagnetic Handbook, by William H. Philpott, W. H. Taplin, and S. Taplin
(Choctaw, OK: Enviro-Tech Products, 1990).
Cross Currents: The Promise of Electromedicine; The Perils of Electropollution, by
Robert O. Becker (New York: Tarcher/Putnam), 1990.
Discovery of Magnetic Health, by George Washins and Richard Hricak
(Rockville, MD: Nove, 1993).
Magnet Therapy: Balancing Your Body's Energy Flow for Self-Healing, by Holger
Hannemann (New York: Sterling, 1990).
The Pain Relief Breakthrough, by Julian Whitaker and Brenda Adderly
(Boston: Little, Brown, 1998).

26

MASSAGE THERAPY

MASSAGE THERAPY IS MUCH MORE than applying oil to sore muscles and rubbing it in. It takes many forms, involves numerous techniques, and ministers to the body in a variety of different ways. While not a cure for diseases, massage in its various forms helps to prevent problems in the body from becoming major issues, at the same time helping to stimulate and revive the body's own healing powers. Since in all matters of health and healing the body is the ultimate hero, it only stands to reason that a therapy like massage that enhances the body's own healing actions should be a vital tool in anyone's cancer-fighting toolbox.

As part of the 11-day Health*Quarters* Lodge program, participants are given three one-hour massages. The benefits and payoffs for each individual are numerous. There are at least two that our guests appreciate most.

STRESS REDUCTION

Stress kills! We all know the saying. But how exactly does stress do this? The American Massage Therapy Association explains it this way:

Stress is an unconscious and automatic reaction to anything we believe may be threatening us. . . . Ideally, this defensive reaction will subside once the situation has resolved, allowing our body to return to its normal state of affairs. However, a person who is frequently under stressful influences will tend to remain locked into a pattern of stress response, unable to relax or let go. This type of pattern is damaging to the body; as it escalates, it ultimately leads to discomfort or pain, and is a contributing factor in most disease processes.[1]

STRENGTHENING IMMUNE FORCES

Read any article about massage therapy and you're bound to find reference made to the Touch Research Institute at the University of Miami School of Medicine. These folks spend their days studying the impact of human touch, and more specifically massage therapy, on human health.

In a recent study, 19 women with either stage 1 or 2 breast cancer were assigned to either a massage therapy group or a control group. Those in the massage group were treated to three 45-minute massages each week for a total of five weeks. At the end of the study, those women who had received the massages showed significantly higher numbers of natural killer cells—the first line of defense in the immune system.[2]

Studies done with HIV-positive men showed the same immune system–enhancing power of massage therapy. Given 45-minute massages five days a week for a month, their numbers of natural killer cells increased.

The conclusion is obvious. Massage should be part of anyone's health battle plan, especially in the case of cancer or AIDS—diseases resulting from a weakened immune system.

ADDITIONAL BENEFITS

Tiffany M. Field, Ph.D., director of the Touch Research Institute, lists other benefits shown in studies on massage therapy:[3]

- Enhanced growth and healthy development in infants, even those who are born prematurely or cocaine- or HIV-exposed

- Reduction of the pain involved in otherwise pain-producing procedures (i.e., childbirth, therapeutic skin brushing of burn victims, recovery from surgery)

- Reduction of the pain levels produced in chronic conditions (i.e., juvenile rheumatoid arthritis, fibromyalgia, lower back pain, migraine headaches, chronic tension headaches)

- Help in addressing mobility problems caused by neuromuscular problems (i.e., multiple sclerosis, spinal cord injuries)

- Enhanced attentiveness and reduction of attention deficits found in autistic children and in those who suffer from attention deficit hyperactivity disorder (ADHD)

- Alleviation of stress, depression, and anxiety

- Lowered blood pressure (in a study of 52 participants who received 15-minute massages at work, there was a significant drop in blood pressure post-massage).

- Help in alleviating much of the stress involved in dealing with autoimmune disorders.

Studies have also shown the beneficial impact of massage on children dealing with diabetes and asthma.

THE RUNDOWN ON RUBDOWNS

The science of massage therapy, as mentioned, takes on many forms and involves a variety of techniques. Since there are so many therapeutic approaches, I describe several that you might run across as you search for a massage therapist to add to your personal health team. You'll find that some therapists are eclectic in their approach—combining a variety of techniques as the need or desire arises. Others prefer to focus their massage work within a limited scope of techniques.

Make massage a vital part of your battle plan. One full body massage every two weeks would be a great place to start. Once a week would be even better if you can afford it.

Aromassage
- The application of plant extracts ("essential oils"—see chapter 23) to provide various effects in combination with massage (for instance: lavender is good for stress reduction, peppermint for fatigue, rosemary for mental stimulation, and sandalwood for creating a romantic mood)

A Few Facts About Massage

- Massage is one of the oldest forms of health-rejuvenating therapy known to man.
- It was first described in China during the second century B.C.
- The word *massage* is derived from the Arabian *mass,* meaning "to press."
- Popularized in the United States in the 1870s by two Swedish doctors, massage became a vital part of medical practice nationwide.
- It was overshadowed in the 1940s with the popularity of pharmaceutical drugs and high-tech medical therapies.
- In 1993 the National Institutes of Health Office of Alternative Medicine allocated funds to study non-mainstream therapies. Of the 30 projects funded, four dealt with massage therapy.

Cranial-sacral
- Mild pressure on various points on the head and neck
- Relieves tension in the face

Deep Tissue
- Also called deep muscle or myofascial or connective tissue
- Similar to Swedish but involves greater pressure to go deeper into tight muscles
- Either follows or goes across grain of muscles, tendons, and fascia
- Goal is to increase range of motion and improve body alignment
- Often used for muscle spasms/scar tissue associated with injuries
- Known to be helpful for those dealing with positional or activity-related discomfort such as carpal-tunnel syndrome

Reflexology
- Also called zone therapy
- Similar to Shiatsu (or acupressure) but is done primarily on the feet and secondarily the hands
- Specific points on the feet and hands are thought to correspond, or "reflex," to all areas of the body via meridians (energy or electricity channels)
- By applying pressure to specific points on the feet or hands, therapists are able to release blocked energy flow in other parts of the body

Shiatsu
- Also called acupressure
- Based on the acupuncture concept that energy/electricity channels, called meridians, run throughout the body
- Therapists open blocked energy flow

Sports
- Another name for "deep tissue" massage
- Targets muscle groups used in specific activity
- Deep tissue pressure
- Used before an event to settle nerves and loosen muscles
- Used after an event to prevent soreness, speed recovery by increasing blood flow, flush lactic acid buildup, stretch muscle tissue

Swedish

- Most common of all the styles
- Characterized by use of long strokes (called effleurage), friction, and kneading on the surface of the muscles
- Oil or powder used on bare skin to smooth therapist's strokes
- Used for relaxation and improvement of circulation

Therapeutic Touch

- Often referred to simply as touch therapy or in some circles the laying on of hands; another form is Reiki
- Not technically a form of massage; no pressure or rubbing involved
- "Healing energy" is transferred to client when therapist places hands on specific areas (the nature of this energy is not fully understood)
- Calming, nurturing

Trigger-point

- Trigger points are defined as especially sensitive nerve bundles that, when compressed by tense muscles, send referred pain to another area of the body. For instance, a headache may be a symptom resulting from muscle spasm originating at a trigger point between the shoulder blades.
- Deep finger pressure applied to points to relieve pain elsewhere

27

ADDITIONAL HELPFUL THERAPIES

ACUPUNCTURE AND ACUPRESSURE

YOU ARE A CHEMICAL BEING made of blood, saliva, urine, stomach acid, and bile. You are also a structural being, with bones, muscles, ligaments, organs, veins and arteries, and skin. Also true, yet often overlooked and underappreciated, is the fact that you are an electrical being.

The heart beats because of an electrical impulse generated within the body. The Chinese recognized long ago the reality of the "body electric." It was they who first determined that energy (electricity) circulates throughout the body along specific channels. They named these channels meridians, and they called the energy *qi* (pronounced "chee"). They also determined that if energy flow along a given meridian was somehow blocked, organs and tissues fed by that particular energy conduit would be adversely affected.

Out of these observations grew the science of acupuncture, the insertion of tiny needles at certain points along meridians to release and enhance energy flow. There are some 360 acupuncture points along the body's 14 major meridians. Acupressure, a related science, is the application of pressure instead of needles at the same acupuncture points along the meridians.

Like any of the other "body strengthening" tools listed in these pages, acupuncture and acupressure don't cure degenerative diseases. There are no such magic bullets. What they can do is to help stimulate your body's own healing powers—which is the ultimate goal when fighting cancer or any other disease process anyhow. If I were in the midst of a cancer battle plan of my own, I'd certainly want an acupuncturist or acupressurist on my personal health team. To find one in your area who meets acceptable standards of competency, you might try contacting this organization:

American Association of Acupuncture and Oriental Medicine
4101 Lake Boone Trail, Suite 201
Raleigh, NC 27607
(919) 787-5181

Another idea is to ask your nutritionist for a referral. Or if all else fails, find an acupuncturist in the yellow pages and give them a try.

CHIROPRACTIC

When it comes to maintaining the body, the brain runs the show. It sends bioelectric messages throughout the body to all its tissues and organs telling them what to do, and it receives messages back in return. The pathways by which these messages are transmitted are the spinal cord and nervous system. We have moving bones of the spine that serve to protect these vulnerable communication pathways. What happens if these bones become misaligned? The result can be disruption in proper communications between the brain and various tissues and organs of the body.

The name for this condition is vertebral subluxation complex: "vertebral," meaning the bones of the spine; "subluxation," meaning less than a total dislocation; "complex," meaning that there is more than just one part. The goal of chiropractic health care is to correct subluxations, thus ensuring that the body is able to continue effectively its self-healing and self-regulating functions.

Studies show that subluxations increase the death rate in humans who are battling pneumonia. Related research shows that spinal care improves the function of the immune system. Since cancer is a disease in which the protective immune system has become compromised, it would seem advantageous to include chiropractic spinal health care in any cancer battle plan.

CHELATION THERAPY

The word "chelation" (pronounced "key-LA-shun") comes from the Greek word "chele," meaning "claw." Chelation therapy is a process in which a solution is introduced into the body by way of an intravenous drip over an extended period of time, usually about three hours, and for a certain number of times, generally 25 to 30 treatments, once or twice a week.

Various ingredients in the solution bind with (or grab onto like a claw) certain undesirable elements that have built up in tissues and along the interior walls of a person's bloodstream. They are then flushed from the system via the kidneys.

The most common solution used as a chelating agent is a blend of the synthetic amino acid ethylene-diamine-tetra-acetic acid (EDTA), with magnesium, B-vitamins, and vitamin C.

What are the "undesirables" that chelation targets? Toxic heavy metals that generate free radicals in the body and in turn damage cells and cause cancer, and abnormal deposits of calcium that help to form health-threatening plaque throughout the circulatory system.

Compared to our ancestors, we all have a whopping excess of toxic heavy metals in our systems—things like mercury, aluminum, cadmium, lead, excessive iron and copper, and others. They enter our bodies from a host of sources: cookware, aluminum cans, seafoods, lead and copper water pipes, exhaust fumes, cooking ingredients, industrial pollutants, dental fillings, tap water, tobacco smoke, animal products, and so on.

In the presence of oxygen, heavy metals such as these stimulate the production of free radicals (wounded molecules) in the body that damage and wound tissues. Cancerous conditions can result.

To find a chelation therapy doctor near you, contact:

American College of Advancement in Medicine (ACAM)
23121 Verdugo Dr., Ste. 204
Laguna Hills, CA 92653
(714) 583-7666
(800) 532-3688 (toll-free outside CA)
www.acam.org

HOMEOPATHY

Homeopathy is a system of stimulating the healing powers of a person's body by using fractionated doses of various substances that in larger doses would actually cause symptoms in a healthy person. It's a concept much like receiving a vaccination—a little bit of the disease being introduced into the body in order to stimulate a response from the immune system to bring about a deep and total cure of that particular illness.

Over the years, more than 1,200 different "like curing like" remedies for various conditions have been identified and cataloged in a work called the Materia Medica, the most important tool of homeopathic health care. These are not drugs, of course, but minute doses ("energy substances") of what would otherwise cause in a healthy person symptoms similar to those being treated in the sick.

Homeopathic remedies are made in a fashion similar to herbal extracts and tinctures but come from a wider variety of sources, including plants, animals, and minerals. Extracts are taken from these various sources and placed individually into what are called mother tinctures. These solutions are then repeatedly diluted and vigorously shaken (potentized).

Oddly enough, the more diluted homeopathic remedies are, the stronger they are. This has to do with quantum physics—the study of vibrational energy. All matter is actually a form of energy. The shaking of the solution releases the energy of the substance into the original tincture, an "energy fingerprint" that stays with the solution and gets more and more potent as it is continually diluted and shaken.

The amount of dilution and potentization is listed on homeopathic remedies by way of letters and numbers.

- "x" or "d" on the bottle means 1 part substance to 9 parts water or alcohol

- "c" means 1 part substance to 99 parts water or alcohol (much more diluted and thus much more potent)

- Numbers before these letters indicate how many times the remedy has been diluted and shaken

Example: a 20c remedy has been diluted and shaken 20 times at a 1 to 99 ratio.

PEELING THE ONION

While the action of allopathic drugs is to drive disease processes deeper into the body's organs and tissues, homeopathy stimulates healing responses in a sick body by responding to "layers" of symptoms until the root cause of the body's illness is reached. It's like peeling an onion.

"In homeopathy," write the editors of *Alternative Medicine,* "the process of healing begins by eliminating the immediate symptoms, then progressing to the older, underlying symptoms. Many of the layers are residues of fevers, trauma, or chronic disease that were unsuccessfully treated or suppressed by conventional medicine."[1]

As this "layer peeling" progresses, it's not unusual for the patient to feel worse before feeling better. This is referred to as a healing crisis. According to the observations made by Dr. Constantine Hering, considered the father of American homeopathy and author of *Hering's Laws of Cure,* such healing progresses from inside the body outward, from the top of the body down, and from the mental/emotional to the physical.

If that's confusing, just remember that homeopathy helps to heal, one layer at a time. If you'll give your body the homeopathic remedies it's asking for right now based on the symptoms it's sending, it will systematically lead you toward the root causes deep beneath other "layers" that are making it sick.

Having homeopathic tinctures available to help stimulate and strengthen your own weakened organs and tissues is an important tool to keep in your cancer-fighting toolbox.

FURTHER READING

Acupuncture and Acupressure

Acupressure Techniques, by Julian Kenyon (Rochester, VT: Healing Arts Press, 1988).

Plain Talk About Acupuncture, by Ellinor R. Mitchell (New York: Whalehall, 1987).

Chelation Therapy

Bypassing Bypass, by Elmer Cranton and Arline Brecher (Hampton Roads, 1990).

Chelation Therapy, by John Parks Trowbridge (Stamford, CT: New Way of Life, 1985).

Homeopathy

The Consumer's Guide to Homeopathy, by Dana Ullman (New York: Tarcher/Putnam), 1995.

Everybody's Guide to Homeopathic Medicines, by Stephen Cummings and Dana Ullman (New York: Tarcher/Putnam, 1991).

Homeopathic Medicine at Home, by Maesimund B. Panos and Jane Heimlich (New York: Tarcher/Putnam), 1980.

ASSESSMENT

TOOLS

You're working hard at winning back your health. You want to know if what you're doing is producing the desired results.

- Is my body getting cleaned out?
- Is the pile of "rocks" getting smaller?
- Is my immune system getting stronger?
- Is my liver sending strong signals?
- Is my digestion what it should be?
- Is my elimination improving?
- Have the parasites been purged?
- Is my thyroid happy?
- Have my nutrient stores increased?
- Am I getting enough fiber?
- Is my dental work still stressing my system?
- Is my cancer going down?

One of the most important things we do at HealthQuarters Lodge is to teach our guests various ways to read how their bodies are doing. We are committed to the concept that God has not only designed our bodies to be self-healing if given the chance but that they communicate in various ways other than words to tell the discerning listener how they're doing.

In the pages that follow are tools for helping to answer the questions listed and more. Some are tools that you can use on yourself, each having its unique contribution to make to the big picture of what you know about your health.

Others require the services of someone trained in their use. How does one tend to find such people? In some cases, for instance with hair analysis, I've been able to give you a phone number at the end of that chapter to call for a referral to a health care professional near you who can help.

Where I am unable to link you with such immediate sources for help, let me suggest the following ideas:

- Yellow pages (local)
- Business card bulletin boards at health food stores
- Health Resources List (available from Health*Quarters* Ministries)

The third item is a list we've compiled over the years (and continue to compile) of various professionals who use nutrition and/or nontoxic therapies to help folks win back their health. This list will not tell you what sort of assessment tools they actually employ in helping people, but in many cases it will give you information on the sorts of therapies they use.

One thing you ought to be aware of before ordering a copy of this list from our office: Health*Quarters* Ministries endorses nobody. In other words, the fact that professionals' names appear on this list does not mean that they necessarily have our seal of approval on their practice. It simply means that we know a bit about what they have to offer and find that they tend to fit into the kind of health care camp we at Home*Quarters* Ministries are part of.

Have fun learning about the assessment tools in the upcoming chapters. When I was first exposed to muscle response testing, I must admit that I was quite skeptical. I had all kinds of questions about this new "weirdness" I was being exposed to. You can read about my experience in *A Cancer Battle Plan*.

Having now studied the science behind it and having been trained in it, I'm daily amazed at the simple tools God has given us to help read these bodies He designed.

If you have questions, feel free to give us a call at Health*Quarters* Ministries: (719) 593-8694.

28

ELECTRODERMAL
SCREENING

THE OTHER DAY I had my son's car towed to the auto repair place. In an attempt to figure out what was wrong, the car mechanics hooked Ben's pride and joy up to a diagnostic computer designed to read the function, or lack thereof, of the various electrical systems necessary to make a car go—he needed a new alternator.

Electrodermal screening (EDS) is a lot like what was done to Ben's car, but in this case it's done to the human body. Long before cars were invented to aid in my illustration, the Chinese discovered, as mentioned earlier, that the body is not just structural and chemical but also electrical. They showed that there are "meridians" running throughout the human system that deliver electrical energy to every organ in the body in order to make the body go.

If somewhere along these lines there is a blockage or disruption of power, the body will not work well. EDS helps to identify and locate these power supply problems.

HOW IS IT DONE?

In electrodermal screening, electrodes are held and/or touched to the body at specific points (acupuncture points along specific meridians being tested), while a device they're connected to (often a computer) measures the electrical skin resistance. The feedback registered gives the practitioner indication of energy blockages or disruptions in various organs and tissues served by the meridian system. The EDS device can then be used to test to see what sort of bioenergetic agent would be helpful to rectify that situation.

Since everything that "is" is made of atoms that have electrons buzzing about them, every food, every vitamin or mineral supplement, and every herb has its own electrical pattern—its own energy. Linking the substance with the point on the body showing weakness, the EDS machine can identify whether or not that particular substance will help to strengthen the particular weakness.

EDS devices can also be used to detect the causes of illnesses such as the presence of bacteria, viruses, parasites, various kinds of chemical toxins, and so on.

WHO INVENTED IT?

In the 1940s, a team of German doctors, under the leadership of an inquisitive medical doctor named Reinhold Voll, proved conclusively that the various places on the body identified by the Chinese as acupuncture points do indeed show a marked decrease in electrical resistance compared to that of the skin around them.

Voll's group also discovered that each point had a standard measurement for anyone who is in good health. As a result of Dr. Voll's work, a number of EDS devices have now been developed, many connected to computers that speed information collecting and categorizing. They are sometimes also referred to as EAV machines (electroacupuncture according to Voll), or electroacupuncture biofeedback devices.

The field of health care that uses electrodermal screening devices is referred to today as energy medicine or bioenergetic medicine. Not only are EDS devices found 'neath this umbrella, but so are muscle response testing and iridology—two assessment tools I enjoy using in my own health ministry with clients (see chapters 29 and 30).

Although health care in the United States has lagged far behind the rest of the world in embracing the concept of the "body electric," the fact is that it's already a well-established part of hospital diagnostics, even if not practiced in the average physician's office. EKG machines measure the electricity of the heart; EEG machines measure brain electricity; Electromyogram (EMG) machines measure electric currents associated with muscle activity. Even the popular magnetic resonance imaging (MRI) machine employs the principles of energy medicine.

ELECTRODERMAL SCREENING AND CANCER

Cancer is a symptom of a body in disrepair, not the cause of the disrepair. People don't die of cancer, they die of the things that allow cancer cells, ever and always present in our bodies, to thrive and multiply. They die of the "rocks." Electrodermal screening, with its ability to identify energy patterns of threats within the body, helps to identify the "rocks"—those things weighing heavily on a body's ability to protect and maintain health. EDS makes getting after the rocks more of an exacting science than a guessing game.

Does that excite you as much as it excites me? EDS truly is the future of cancer therapy and health care in general in the United States. Imagine every doctor's office equipped with an EDS device so that, just like towing your ailing car in for a test, you could haul your aching body in for a complete diagnostic in order to identify and target the causes of your cancerous condition.

EDS, where it is now being used, not only helps to design game plans for treating bodies fighting cancer but also helps prevent its onset in the first place.

FURTHER READING

Alternative Medicine, by the Burton Goldberg Group (Tiburon, CA: Future Medicine, 1993), pages 192–204.

"Basic Explanation of the Electrodermal Screening Test and the Concepts of Bio-Energetic Medicine," by the American Association of Acupuncture and Bioenergetic Medicine. (On the Internet at www.healthy.net/pan/pa/aaabem/EAV/eavexplained.htm)

"The Past, Present, and Future of the Electrodermal Screening System (EDSS)," by Julia J. Tsuei, *Journal of Advancement in Medicine,* Winter 1995. (On the Internet at www.healthy.net/pan/pa/aaabem/pastpresent/index.html)

MUSCLE RESPONSE TESTING

EVERY ORGAN AND TISSUE in the body is bioenergetic—it emits an energy pattern. As discussed in the last chapter, it is possible, using an electrodermal screening device, to measure such energy as an indication of the health or lack thereof of that particular body part or system. However, even without the aid of such a device, it is still possible to ascertain which parts of the body are weak and asking for assistance and which are strong.

If you've not already read the previous chapter on electrodermal screening, do so first before reading further. Muscle response testing (MRT)—sometimes referred to as kinesiology—is much like electrodermal screening, but without a device.

Let's suppose you came to Health*Quarters* Ministries for a nutritional assessment. Using muscle response testing, the first thing I'd do is get a feel for your relative muscle strength. Having you make a circle by bringing the tip of your thumb to the tip of your middle finger, I'd ask you to resist as I tried to pull them apart.

The key here is that this is not a wrestling match. As the tester, my goal is to gauge the other individual's relative strength. What is the level of the person's strongest response to my challenge of his or her finger muscles?

Many who use MRT will challenge the shoulder muscle instead of the fingers. They do this by having their client hold one arm out parallel to the floor, locking the shoulder muscle in place. Wrapping one hand around the client's outstretched wrist, the tester then gently but firmly presses downward, gauging the relative strength of that muscle.

Once I've gotten a feel for your relative strength, I want to see if the electrical system in your body is flowing well and is testable or whether there is some sort of interference that must first be dealt with.

First I'll have you put your left hand, palm down, on top of your head, having you once again make the circle with thumb and middle finger on your right hand, and resisting my pull on that connection. That right-hand connection should remain strong.

Then I'll have you flip your left hand over so that it is palm up on the top of your head, and once again I'll challenge the right-hand finger connection. If your electrical system is unblocked and flowing well, the right-hand finger connection should now be weak.

Why, you ask?

We have a north magnetic pole (our head) and a south magnetic pole (our feet). Correspondingly, the top of the hand is north, and the bottom is south. When the palm is flat against the top of the head, you've made a south/north magnetic connection. Opposites poles attract. The electrical flow through your body remains uninterrupted. The muscle in the right-hand finger connection remains strong.

However, when you flipped that left hand over on the top of your head, you put a north pole to a north pole. These repel each other, interrupting the electrical flow through your body, and should result in a weakening of the finger connection being tested on the right hand.

In the event that in the north-on-north position (back of the left hand to top of head) your right-hand finger connection is still strong, that's a signal that something is blocking or disrupting the proper electrical flow in your body.

Anything electrical being worn on the body may be the cause of interrupted electrical flow (a good reason not to wear battery-run watches, beepers, cell phones, etc.). After removing these, retesting may well get the north-on-north weakness I'm looking for. If not, a second remedy would be to have you drink a glass of water. The proper electrical flow in our bodies is dependent on sufficient amounts of H_2O in the system. Unfortunately, most of us are chronically and persistently dehydrated.

If after the water your right-hand finger connection is still testing strong to that north/north connection atop your head, the next thing I'll try is to have you put some magnesium capsules in your pocket. Most Americans are mineral deficient. In fact aging is the "demineralization" of the body. Without sufficient mineral supplies, electrical flow is hindered. The mineral the majority of Americans need most and get least is magnesium.

OK, let's suppose that we've now gotten you to the point where your north-on-north position brings a weak response to the finger connection. And let's suppose that I now want to check to see how your liver is doing. What I'll do is have you hold the palm of your left hand against the ribs at the base of your right rib cage. Your liver resides in that area. Testing your right-hand finger connection for strength will now tell me if your liver is sending a weak or strong signal.

In similar fashion we could check all your organs, tissues, and various nutrient stores in your body in a matter of just a few minutes. Thus MRT is a "low tech, high touch," inexpensive, fun, and easily learned tool for gathering a fairly accurate picture about the strengths and weaknesses of your system.

With MRT, the practitioner is not diagnosing diseases but looking for weaknesses, with the thought that ministering nutrition to those weaknesses will help the body work as a whole better and thus conquer whatever ails it. It's a wonderful tool for those of us who believe that God designed the body to be self-protective and self-healing if given a chance and that the only cure to cancer or any other degenerative disease is the good working of the body.

MINISTERING TO NUTRITIONAL WEAKNESSES

Your liver sent a weak signal. How do you minister nutritionally to it? I have a test kit consisting of nutritional supplements. When it comes to nutrition for the liver, I've got on hand half a dozen different herbal blends that are known to minister to liver weakness.

I'll pull one from the kit and have you hold it to your liver with your left hand, and I'll test the right-hand finger connection. A strong response means it would help to strengthen your liver. You see, whatever is in that little bottle has its own electrical energy, since all things that "are" are made of atoms with electrons whizzing about them. If the electrical energy of that substance makes the liver's energy strong, that's what you're looking for.

Wherever we found weakness in your system, we'd follow a similar pattern of testing. For each area of the body I test, I have several different products on hand (mostly herbs) that have been historically known to minister to nutritional deficiencies found there. I simply test until I find one that works, and I go with that.

As to the amount to take, having you hold a few capsules in your closed left hand against your stomach while I test your right-hand finger connection will give an idea of how many a day your body would value. I usually start with six. If that's too many, the right-hand finger connection will be weak. I'll take one away until I get a strong response. If the response is strong with six, I'll keep adding capsules until I get a weak response, then take one away.

IDENTIFYING FOOD ALLERGIES

Another fascinating thing about MRT is its use in helping folks know what sort of foods they might be allergic to, or at least have a hard time digesting. By having you hold different substances next to your stomach, we can determine which are the ones that make your right-hand finger connection weak and thus should be avoided.

I carry about 30 different foods in my kit. Those to which clients are universally weak are sugar and dairy. These are not so much allergy foods as things that are hard on the human body. With dairy, most of us simply do not have the enzyme needed (lactase) to break down the sugars in dairy (lactose).

Foods to which folks are often actually allergic include the grains, particularly wheat. Usually as people go through the "unloading" of toxic waste from their systems, they tend to regain the ability to eat the kinds of foods that may have once caused an allergic response in their system. When an allergen is consumed, the body produces excess mucus to protect its "innards" from the offending substance. Although food allergies will not always or even often result in an outward manifestation of trouble, they certainly can be troublesome internally as mucus builds up.

FOR YOUR INFORMATION

A sample checklist follows that you can use with MRT to do a nutritional assessment. Let me encourage you to practice on your family and friends, making it your goal to become knowledgeable with this assessment tool.

Remember, have your client put a finger or palm of the left hand on the various "touch points" while you muscle test the right–hand finger connection (tip of thumb to tip of middle finger). If there is a weakness, you may wish to get the recommended product and test to see if it makes the test point strong. I keep several products in my test kit matched to each touch point; here I'm only listing one for space reasons. Many of these supplements are available at your local health food store. They can also be ordered from Health*Quarters* Ministries.

Test	Touch Point	Potential Product
Blood pressure	Index finger on top of head	GC-X
Pituitary	Index finger at top of hair line/forehead	Pro-Gest cream
Protein	Twist little hairs at base of scalp	Spirulina
Stress	Palm of hand on forehead	Nutri-calm
Pineal gland	Squeeze bridge of nose with thumb and index finger	GG-C
Vitamin A	Index finger to right eyelid shut	Spirulina
Respiratory allergies	Pinch membrane between nostrils	Whole System Thymus
Food allergies	Finger below center of bottom lip	(Check which foods)
Thymus	Tap halfway down sternum	Whole System Thymus
Lymph	Touch-tap behind jaw/below ear	Whole System Thymus
Potassium	Hollow of right cheek	Potassium Combination
Sodium	Hollow of left cheek	BP-X
RNA/DNA	Four fingers across base of hair line	Spirulina
Thyroid	Middle finger in sternal notch with forefinger and ring finger either side of Adam's apple	KC-X
Trace minerals	Left side of neck on sterno-cleidomastoid muscle even with Adam's apple	Three (contains kelp, dandelion, alfalfa)
Vitamin E	Below outer half of collarbone on right side	Three

Test	Touch Point	Potential Product
Vitamin F	Soft spot inside end of right collarbone next to neck	Red raspberry
Calcium	Above inside end of left collarbone next to neck	CA Herbal
Vitamin C	Below outer half of collarbone on left side	Red raspberry
Lungs	Tap/hold outer rib cage 2 inches below collarbone, either side	ALJ
Heart/circulation	3 inches below collarbone, both sides	HS II
Hydrochloric acid	1 inch below sternum on angle of ribs, left side	Food enzymes
Enzymes	Same as above, but on right side	Food enzymes
Acidophilus	1½ inches below enzyme point on rib, right side	PB8
Gallbladder	Base of rib cage, right side	Food enzymes
Liver	2 inches above gallbladder point	Liv-A
Zinc	Inside crest of right hip bone	Spirulina
Iron	At pants crease where right leg meets torso	Liv-A
Vitamin D	At pants crease where left leg meets torso	Red raspberry
Copper/phosphorus	Inside crest of left hip bone	Gotu kola
Parasites	Tip of left thumb to little finger	Para-Cleanse
Yeast	Tip of left thumb to ring finger	PB8
Virus	One finger 1 inch below navel	IGS II
Magnesium malate	1 inch below navel, three fingers spread horizontally	Magnesium
Heavy metals	One finger on top of pubic bone	Kelp
Bladder	1 inch above pubic bone on midline of body	K
Prostate	2 inches above pubic bone Three fingers placed horizontally	X-A
Ovaries/uterus	(Same as prostate)	Pro-Gest

Test	Touch Point	Potential Product
Colon	Tap vertically halfway between hip and navel, horizontally above navel	Perfect 7
Kidneys	On back, 4 inches base of ribs	K
Adrenals	2 inches above navel, one finger	New Image Plus
Pancreas	One finger below left rib cage, thumb to shirt seam	New Image Plus
Joints	Place palm over area	JNT-A
Dental	Place finger along all four tooth lines, test each individually	See biological dentist

FURTHER READING

The Ultimate Healing System, by Donald Lepore (Woodland, 1985).

Your Body Can Talk, by Susan L. Levy and Carol Lehr (Prescott, AZ: HOHM Press), 1996.

Your Body Doesn't Lie, by John Diamond (New York: Warner, 1979).

IRIDOLOGY

IRIDOLOGY IS THE SCIENCE of studying the effects of electrical impulses on the iris of the eye. The iris is the most highly specialized nerve organ in your whole body, with the most highly developed nerve tissue. All electrical impulses sent forth by all organs and tissues leave their mark on the iris. The iris is to the body what the TV screen is to television broadcasting—a receiver of the signal.

Over the 150 years that the science of iridology has existed, doctors and scientists who have studied it have correlated a specific area of the iris with each major organ and tissue in the body. In other words, the electrical impulses being sent forth by that organ or tissue are reflected in a specific part of the iris. (See *Iridology Simplified,* by Bernard Jensen.)

The vibratory signals sent forth by your stomach always show themselves in a certain part of the iris—so too, the intestines, the thyroid, kidneys, lungs, brain, and so on. It's easy to locate the stomach and the intestines on the chart on page 205. They are always found within the first area encircling the pupil, which is the center of the iris. Other organs or tissues can be easily located by using the number ring located around the outer rim of the iris on the chart. It corresponds to a clock face. For instance, the kidneys are found at 32 minutes in the left iris and 27 minutes in the right.

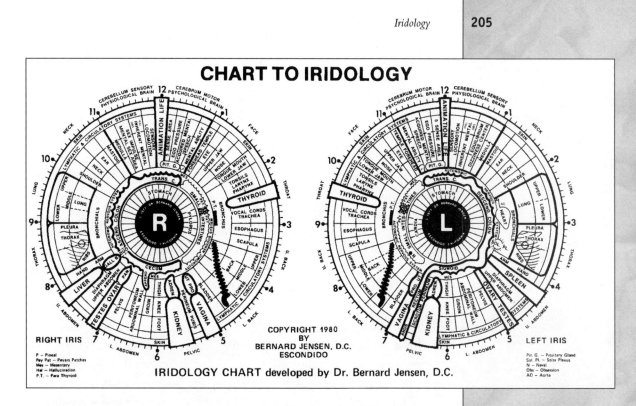

CHART TO IRIDOLOGY

RIGHT IRIS

P — Pineal
Pey Pat — Peyers Patches
Mes — Mesentery
Hal — Hallucination
P.T. — Para Thyroid

COPYRIGHT 1980
BY
BERNARD JENSEN, D.C.
ESCONDIDO

LEFT IRIS

Pit. G. — Pituitary Gland
Sol. Pl. — Solar Plexus
N — Naval
Obs — Obsession
AO — Aorta

IRIDOLOGY CHART developed by Dr. Bernard Jensen, D.C.

It has also been well established that all organs and tissues on the right side of the body will present themselves in the right iris. Likewise, the left side of the body will show in the left iris. For instance, there are two kidneys, one on each side of the body. The left one shows in the left iris; the right one shows in the right. The heart, an organ located only in the left side of the body, will have its electrical vibrations received and reflected in the left iris only. Similarly, the liver, a right-side-of-the-body organ, shows only in the right iris.

Observing the iris locations of various organs and tissues, the person trained in this science can identify by the coloration or markings found at those points how the corresponding parts of the body are doing. A brown spot found in any organ area could well mean a buildup of toxic material or drug deposits in that organ. Certain things could then be done to minister to and strengthen the organ. Such spots are called psora (pronounced "sora").

A lesion, technically known as a lacuna, is another sign a trained iridologist will look for in the iris. The fibers of the eye in good health will be tightly packed, like the pages of a closed book. Lacunae are openings in these fibers that look like the pages of a wet book. The darker the area within the lacuna, the more degenerated is the organ or tissue being represented. As things are done to minister to this area of weakness, healing signs will appear—white fiber lines that make a crisscross pattern in the open lesion. This is an indication of healing and cleansing.

A FEW "EYE SIGNS" FOR THE BEGINNER

There are actually quite a number of potential markings or colorations one might find at any one organ or tissue location in the iris. Each sends its own message as to the vitality of that member of the body. However, lest I get too complex, I'll present just seven "eye signs" to get you started. A penlight shone into the eye from the side, while viewing the iris with a magnifying glass, is the best way to practice this sort of detective work. Do this to a friend, then have him or her do it for you.

Lymphatic Rosary

This is characterized by a ring of tiny white, or discolored, "clouds" located near the outer rim of the iris. It is an indication that the lymph system—the garbage collection system in the body—is loaded with toxic buildup. A person with this sign (and by the way, any of these seven can appear in either or both eyes) will probably have problems with mucus buildup in the body, such as sinus congestion, asthma, swollen lymph nodes, frequent colds, and a predisposition to kidney problems.

Remedies

1. Herbs that increase lymph flow: yarrow, capsicum, lobelia, echinacea, Oregon grape, ginger, horseradish

2. Exercise is essential; rebounding (see chapter 16) is considered the best form of exercise for stimulating lymph drainage

3. Dry skin brushing (see chapter 14)

4. Deep breathing (see chapter 9)

5. Avoid dairy products and other mucus-producing foods (meat of all kinds, grains of all kinds unless sprouted)

Nerve Rings

Observable rings that travel all or part way around the interior of the iris are indicative of neuromuscular tension and stress in the body. Find the location of the nerve rings on the iridology chart. The organ locations that are transversed by these rings reveal which parts of your body are taking the most abuse from the tension and stress.

Remedies

1. Herbs that soothe and build the nervous system: chamomile, passion flower, valerian root, hops, lobelia, horsetail, skullcap; STR-J formula from NSP (contains chamomile, passion flower, fennel, feverfew, hops and marshmallow); Nutri-Calm formula from NSP (blend of B-vitamins with hops, passion flower, valerian root, and several other synergistic herbs)

2. Calcium and magnesium supplements

3. Deep tissue massage

4. Feed the thyroid with kelp

5. Resolve emotional stress

Radii Solaris (Parasite Lines)

These lines look like the spokes of a bicycle wheel radiating outward from the pupil area. They are a sign that the nervous system is weak, or has been weakened, allowing for toxic buildup and parasitic activity in the colon. This isn't the only eye sign that might lead one to consider the presence of parasites, but it is a pretty clear indication of that possibility.

Remedies

1. Products to improve digestion and elimination and to kill the parasites (see chapter 17)

2. Herbs that soothe the nervous system (the same as listed for the nerve rings)

3. Colon cleansing (see chapter 18)

Stomach Halo

This is a round, white or gray ring that surrounds the pupil. It is usually a sign of digestive problems, sometimes of the presence of a hiatal hernia. When the ring is bright white, it's a sign that the stomach is making too much digestive acid—otherwise known as hydrochloric acid (HCl). The reality is, however, that as we age we tend to make less and less. The bloating, gas, and indigestion problems so often medicated with TV-promoted antacid products actually do not address the issue. The same conditions arise when a person's stomach is not making enough acid to break down foods. Antacids used in this situation simply tell the stomach to quit trying and pass the food on to the intestines. The problem, the lack of digestive power, is never addressed. What might be described as a "dirty" or grayish-white ring is an indication of underacidity.

Remedies

1. White: overactive production of hydrochloric acid

   Herbs to slow production: Fennel, yucca root, slippery elm, catnip

   Sodium foods: celery, carrots, cabbage, parsley, dandelion greens

2. Dark: underactive production of hydrochloric acid

   Food enzymes from NSP to help digestion

   B-vitamins to help production of hydrochloric acid

   Acidophilus to help body's production of B-vitamins

Scurf Rim

If there's a darkened rim around the outside of the iris, that's a scurf rim. This sign is indicative of underactive or weakened tendencies of the skin. Our bodies have been designed to sweat—to eliminate, on the average, two pounds of toxic waste each day. When, for whatever reason, our skin is underactive, often a buildup of toxic waste takes place in the bowel and lungs that is hard to get rid of.

Remedies

1. Herbs to enhance skin health (high in silica): horsetail, dulse

2. Dry skin brushing (see chapter 14)

3. Sweat baths

   - Epsom salt soak: 2 lbs. in tub of hot water for 30 minutes while drinking cold water

   - Herbal soak: ½ teaspoon ginger mixed in the tub of hot water with 1 cup apple cider vinegar; soak for 30 minutes while drinking cold water

4. Sauna: dry sauna is an excellent way to work up a sweat; don't use steamrooms; breathing in all that chlorine from chlorinated water will be counterproductive to your efforts to detoxify

5. Exercise (a must)

6. Niacin (B3) with exercise (start with 100 milligrams)

Lipid or Sodium/Cholesterol Ring

This is the name given to a cloudy ring around all or part of the outer edge of the iris. It appears to overlay the eye fibers, partially hiding them—like looking through murky water at something at the bottom of the sink. This is a sign associated with calcium, cholesterol, and/or fatty deposits in the body. The correlation between this cloudiness and middle-age death from heart disease or stroke is strong. It also can indicate that there are problems with the liver and thyroid and increased risk for diabetes and Parkinson's disease. Closely related to this sign is the condition of cataracts, which are formed by calcium falling out of solution and settling in the lens of the eye. The same free-floating calcium can lead to hardening of arteries affecting other organs, such as the ears and hearing.

Remedies

1. Herbs to cleanse and build the blood: hawthorn, capsicum, garlic, butcher's broom; BP-X formula from NSP (contains burdock, pau d'arco, red clover, sarsaparilla, yellow dock, dandelion, buckthorn, cascara sagrada, peach bark, yarrow, Oregon grape, prickly ash)

2. Herbs to cleanse and build the liver: milk thistle, burdock, uva ursi, yucca; LIV-A formula from NSP (contains red beet, dandelion, parsley, horsetail, yellow dock, black cohosh, birch, blessed thistle, angelica, chamomile, gentian, goldenrod); milk thistle combination formula from NSP

3. Coffee retention enemas to stimulate the liver to purge itself (see chapter 18)

4. Avoidance of saturated fats and cholesterol in diet

5. Herbs rich in organic sodium to deal with calcium deposits: hydrangea, parsley, dandelion, eyebright

6. Chelation therapy: a series of intravenous drips administered by a doctor and done over a period of days or weeks, aimed at helping to remove plaque buildup from arteries

7. Oral chelation (I like to suggest the use of a product called MegaChel from NSP)

Arcus Sinilus

In this condition the top of the iris looks like it's actually fading away. This sign (seen most in the elderly) is an indication that the brain is not experiencing adequate circulation. As we age, those members of our body above our heart tend to get less blood supplied to them. If the brain is not getting enough oxygen and nutrients because of reduced blood supply, there is a tendency toward senility, absentmindedness, poor memory, and sleepiness while sitting.

Remedies

1. Herbs that improve circulation to the brain: ginkgo biloba, gotu kola, capsicum; GGC formula from NSP—(contains capsicum, Siberian ginseng, gotu, kola); MindMax, a liquid herb preparation from NSP (contains gingko biloba, Korean ginseng, gotu kola)

2. Exercise

Many of the products listed here are available at your local health food store or from your nutrition professional. They can also be ordered from Health*Quarters* Ministries.

FURTHER READING

Iridology Simplified, by Bernard Jensen (Escondido, CA: Bernard Jensen, 1980).

The Science and Practice of Iridology, by Bernard Jensen, vol. 1 (Escondido, CA: Bernard Jensen, 1995).

31

THE AMAS
BLOOD TEST

THE ANTIMALIGNIN ANTIBODY IN AERUM (AMAS for short) blood test is designed to measure the amount of antibodies your system is manufacturing for the fight. A measure of this "ammunition" is an indication of the size of the enemy force the body is facing.

We've all got cancer in our bodies—at least cancer cells. As I've previously pointed out, at any one time the average American has up to 10,000 cancer cells floating around in his or her system. The goal is to keep the body's protective mechanisms strong against these rebel cells so that they can't get organized and create tumors. As a protective measure against cancer cells in the system, the body manufactures things called antibodies. Their job is to seek out and destroy foreign proteins, chief of which are cancer cells.

In other words, the AMAS test has the potential to tell you at what level cancer is present in your body.

TEST CHARACTERISTICS

The AMAS is a general cancer test, independent of cell type.
The AMAS test has the potential to tell you whether or not there is cancer

actively growing in your body, but it can't tell you where. It's a measure of what the body is doing to fight cancer cells, regardless of where they are located. That may seem frustrating to some. I mean, after all, wouldn't a person want to know where his or her cancer is growing?

Remember that your body is the hero. The only cure to cancer, or any other disease for that matter, is your body itself. The whole point of this book is to help you learn how to build and restore your body's fighting power, as opposed to simply attacking the symptom. Cancerous growths are symptoms of a whole system that is not working well.

Where such thinking prevails, the AMAS test can be extremely helpful to see if the things you're doing to help the body rebuild are working. Does this mean that other blood tests should not be pursued? Antigen tests like the carcino-embryonic antigen, prostate specific antigen, and carcinoma 125? No, they too can be potentially helpful. They measure the amount of protein being released into the bloodstream by a cancerous growth. When the counts go up, it's assumed the cancer is growing.

I say "assumed" because it's not always true that rising counts are a sign of growing cancer activity. When the body's fighting forces are strengthened by way of the types of therapies presented in this book, their goal will be to break apart and destroy the tumor. The bloodstream will be flooded with the same proteins for removal that might otherwise be read as a sharp increase in cancer growth. Bottom line, when you're taking the approach of building the body so that it can cure the cancer, the AMAS test (measuring antibodies) may prove more appropriate and less confusing than measuring antigens.

The AMAS test has lower false positive and false negative rates than antigen tests and is often elevated earlier.

One would hope that any and all tests would be accurate and helpful 100 percent of the time. This, however, is true of no test—not even the AMAS. Nevertheless, the AMAS test has been shown to be 95 percent accurate upon initial use, growing to 99 percent accuracy if the test is repeated to verify results.[1]

AMAS test results are elevated when the level of malignant cells present in the body is elevated, returning to within the normal range when the number of malignant cells is reduced. When test results are returned, a range is given. If you fall between 0 and 99, that means your body does indeed have cancer cells, as most bodies do, but it would appear that you don't have a cancerous process going on. If you fall between 100 and 134, you probably have a cancerous process going on. At 135 or above, it's a sure bet that you do have a cancerous process happening in your system.

The AMAS test is especially helpful for folks at high risk for developing cancer. This would include:

1. Those who have already experienced the disease

2. Those who have a family history of cancer

3. Those who have been exposed to known carcinogens (cancer-causing agents)

4. Those who are over 50 years of age

The AMAS test doesn't work well for folks whose bodies are already so compromised by disease that they are simply not making any antibodies.
This tends to be people for whom cancer has reached an advanced or clearly "terminal" state. In such a situation, the AMAS test reading will not be elevated even though there is significant cancerous growth.

The AMAS test is covered by Medicare and thus may be reimbursable by your insurance company.
Your doctor may have no knowledge of this test since those who designed it do no advertising. It has, however, been available for many years and has been written about in the *New England Journal of Medicine*. Additional information concerning the AMAS test can be found in the reading list for this chapter.

Steps to Completing the Test

1. You or your doctor calls the one lab in the country that does this test. Request that an AMAS test kit be sent either directly to you or to your doctor's office. Minimal cost, if any, is involved in having the kit sent.

2. You will need to have blood drawn and processed according to the detailed instructions accompanying the kit. If your doctor's office is unable to do this, they'll send you to a local lab for that purpose.

3. After the blood is drawn and processed per instructions, it must be packed in dry ice in the test kit container and sent overnight with the appropriate paperwork signed (comes with kit) and with a check for payment ($210 at the time of this writing). (You may have to bring dry ice with you to the lab unless they have it available there.)

4. You will receive back a simple one-page report with a number on it that shows within what range your body is developing antibodies to fight cancer, which will in turn signal the extent to which cancer may be active in your body.

Only one lab in the country does the actual AMAS test on blood samples:

Oncolab, Inc.
36 The Fenway
Boston, MA 02215
1(800) 9CA-TEST
(617) 536-0657 (FAX)

THE AMAS TEST VERSUS MAMMOGRAPHY

The track record for mammography is not good. On any given day 20 to 30 percent of women getting them receive back false negatives (told there's nothing to worry about when really there is), while another 20 to 30 percent are given a false positive (told there's cancer present when really there isn't). This means that for every 10 women getting a mammogram, 6 will end up with inaccurate information concerning the true condition of their breast tissues.[2]

Were I a woman, I would never subject myself to mammography. Not only is accuracy an issue, so is the radiation involved. There is no safe level of exposure. The AMAS test would be my choice.

To all who are fighting cancer, let me suggest that you investigate the AMAS test. It will help you establish a baseline of feedback as to how your body is currently doing against cancer cells. Then as you work your way through the cleansing and strengthening battle plan outlined in this book, periodically redo the test (perhaps every three months) to see how your body is responding to the help you're giving it.

SOURCES FOR MORE INFORMATION ABOUT THE AMAS TEST

Alternative Medicine Guide to Women's Health 2, by Burton Goldberg and the editors of *Alternative Medicine* (Tiburon, CA: Future Medicine, 1998).
Definitive Guide to Cancer, by W. John Diamond and W. Lee Cowden with Burton Goldberg (Tiburon, CA: Future Medicine, 1997).

32

DARK FIELD MICROSCOPY (A.K.A. LIVE BLOOD ANALYSIS)

DARK FIELD MICROSCOPY, also referred to as live cell analysis or live blood analysis, is a relatively new assessment tool. It used to be that the only way to view blood was by using electron microscopes, which subjected the blood sample to the effects of both vacuum and electrons, the impact of which made it "virtually impossible to observe living organisms" in the blood.[1]

I had the privilege of having a drop of blood drawn from my finger and examined under considerable magnification using what is called a dark field microscope. It was wired to a monitor that received images of what was happening inside that drop of my liquid life. I saw life in action inside my bloodstream.

Being able to actually view the activity levels of various things at work in your bloodstream is of extraordinary value. Whereas the electron microscope simply allowed for a counting-up of the number of white blood cells present in the sample, the dark field microscope allows the viewer to actually assess the white blood cells' health and functional capability as they chase after (or don't) the things they're supposed to be killing.

A practitioner trained in this living blood analysis can identify a multitude of things, including:

- Red blood cell health and oxygen-carrying ability
- White blood cell health and count
- Hormone imbalances
- Glandular abnormalities
- Presence of plaque and cardiac by-products
- Bowel and liver toxicity levels and damage
- Vitamin and mineral status and deficiencies
- Enzyme needs
- Oxygenation levels
- Extent of free radical damage to cells
- Blood clotting capability
- Cholesterol and tryglyceride excesses
- Tendencies toward allergies
- Tendencies toward disease processes
- Bacterial presence
- Yeast presence
- Parasite presence

I suddenly became extra motivated to do regular parasite purgings when I saw mine on the screen (see chapter 17). Based on what is seen, the practitioner is able to accurately put together a program of diet changes, nutritional supplements, and perhaps other sorts of herbal and nutritional agents all aimed at ministering to the specific need. Pictures can be recorded to view at a later date to see if progress has been made toward specific goals.

Concerning the use of this sort of assessment tool in his own practice, Douglas Brodie, M.D., of Reno, Nevada, says: "In many cases, the live blood analysis provides information that enables us to predict which direction the cancer patient's body is heading. We then make specific adjustments in nutrition and other modalities to optimize the healing process."[2]

HOW TO FIND SOMEONE NEAR YOU WHO
DOES DARK FIELD MICROSCOPY

A key pioneer of this assessment tool is James R. Privitera, M.D. He is the director of NutriScreen, Inc, of Covina, California, where he is in private practice in allergy and nutrition. His affiliations include the American Preventive Medical Association, the International College of Applied Nutrition, and the National Health Federation.

If you have problems locating someone near you who uses dark field microscopy, Dr. Privitera's office may be able to point you in the right direction. Their toll free number as of this writing is 1-888-220-7888.

FURTHER READING

Silent Clots: Life's Biggest Killers, by James R. Privitera and Alan Stang (Encino, CA: Catacombs Press, 1995).

HAIR, FINGERNAIL, AND TONGUE OBSERVATIONS

YOUR HAIR TELLS A STORY

THE GROWING HAIR FOLLICLE is richly supplied with blood vessels, and the blood that bathes the follicle is the transport medium for both essential and potentially toxic elements. These elements are then incorporated into the growing hair protein. . . . Thus, element concentrations of the hair reflect concentrations in other body tissues.[1]

Thus say scientists at Great Smokies Diagnostic Laboratory (GSDL) in Asheville, North Carolina.

Analysis of hair samples taken from a person's head can reveal the level of nutrient minerals being absorbed from food into the person's bloodstream. It can also reveal the level of exposure a person is receiving to toxins.

HAIR ANALYSIS AND DETOXIFICATION

From my point of view, the most valuable aspect of hair analysis is what it can tell us about the "rocks" we may have accumulated in our bodies that are weighing heavily against their ability to maintain health.

We're being exposed daily to various levels of toxic metals. These include things like mercury from dental fillings and seafood; lead from water pipes and gasoline products; aluminum from cans, cookware, and antiperspirants; nickel from stainless-steel pots and pans; and on and on. We know without a doubt that toxic heavy metals such as these weigh heavily against the body's protective immune system.

Hair analysis is a great tool for discovering the levels at which these things have gathered in our tissues and thus what part they have played in the onset of a disease process. Concentrations of these toxins can be up to three hundred times higher in hair than what might appear in a blood test or urine sample.

In any war it's of fundamental importance to know the enemy. In cancer, the enemy is not the cancer cell but the thing or things that allowed it to proliferate. Hair analysis, then, can help to identify the targets at which the cancer warrior needs to aim his or her detoxing tools.

WHERE TO FIND HELP

For a referral to a health care professional near you who can accomplish this testing for you, call the Great Smokies Diagnostic Lab at 1-800-522-4762. I'm a great fan of GSDL, as you can no doubt tell. They're at the core of what is called functional medicine—a focus on the function of various organs and systems in the body as opposed to focusing on disease processes. Get all things working together in the body as they should, and the body will cure the disease.

FINGERNAIL OBSERVATIONS

It has long been known that a careful examination of one's fingernails can give some solid clues concerning the quality of the inner workings of the body if you know what you're looking for.

To the informed observer these clues can function as warning signs. In her book *Healthy Healing,* Linda Rector-Page, N.D., Ph.D., observes that the nails "are one of the last tissues to receive the nutrients carried by the blood, and show signs of trouble before other better-nourished tissues do."[2]

On the other hand, an improvement in fingernail health may serve to send notice that the things you're doing to try to win back your health are actually working. Checking them thoroughly once a week can be part of a disciplined approach to keeping in touch with what's happening in your body.

Nail Signals	Potential Message (any or all may apply)
Color	
Greenish	Internal bacteria infection Localized fungal infection
Yellow	Lymphatic problems Respiratory problems Diabetes Liver disorders Vitamin E deficiency Poor circulation
Dark or discolored	B12 deficiency Anemia Liver problems Kidney problems
White (pale, without luster)	Liver disorder Kidney disorder Anemia General mineral deficiency "Blood vacuity"—lack of life force
White (waxy)	Ulcerative bleeding Hookworm or other parasitical infestation
White spots	Thyroid problem Zinc deficiency Calcium deficiency Parasitical infestation HCl (hydrochloric acid) deficiency Chronic constipation Fatigue
White with pink near tips	Cirrhosis
White with round dot (left middle finger)	Diabetes
Half white with dark spots at tip	Kidney disease

Nail Signals	Potential Message (any or all may apply)
Color	
White lines	Heart disease High fever Arsenic poisoning
White lines (single, horizontal)	Liver disease Lead poisoning Arsenic poisoning
Two white horizontal bands that do not move as nail grows	Hypoalbuminemia (protein deficiency in blood)
Deep blue beds	Pulmonary obstructive disorder (asthma, emphysema) Lung and heart problems Drug reaction Blood toxicity (too much silver or copper)
Dark blue band in bed	Skin cancer (especially in the light-skinned)
White dumbbell shape in center of left ring fingernail (nail may also be red/purplish)	Prostate problems
White crescent shape in lower right corner of left ring finger nail	Uterine fibroids
Red moon	Heart problems
Slate blue moon	Heavy metal poisoning Lung problems
Red skin around cuticles	Poor metabolism of essential fatty acids Connective tissue disorder (lupus, etc.)
Black, splinterlike bits beneath	Infectious endocarditis (heart infection) Heart disease Bleeding disorder
Black bands	Chemotherapy reaction Radiation reaction
Clouded, opaque	Candida (systemic yeast infection)

Nail Signals	Potential Message (any or all may apply)
Contour	
Downward curved ends	Heart problems Liver problems Respiratory problems
Broaden at tip and curve downwards	Lung damage (emphysema, asbestos, etc.)
Flat	Raynaud's disease—insufficient oxygen in bloodstream resulting in discoloration of hands (white or blue) Low disease resistance/ physical weakness
Thin, flat, spoon-shaped	B12 deficiency Anemia
Raised base, with small, white ends	Respiratory disorder (emphysema, chronic bronchitis, etc.)
Elevation of tip	Lymphatic problems Respiratory problems Diabetes Liver disorders
Unusually wide, square	Hormonal disorder
Grooves (vertical)	Poor general health Poor nutrient absorption Iron deficiency Kidney disorder Tendency to develop arthritis Vitamin A deficiency Protein deficiency Calcium deficiency
Grooves (horizontal)	Severe emotional/psychological stress Severe physical stress (infection, disease, intestinal parasites) Chronic intestinal weakness
Horizontal groove (index finger)	Tendency to develop skin diseases
Horizontal groove (ring finger)	Eye problems Bronchitis Respiratory disease
Horizontal groove (middle finger)	Associated with loss of muscle strength

Nail Signals	Potential Message (any or all may apply)
Contour	
Horizontal groove (little finger)	Throat problems Nerve disorders Gallbladder troubles
Horizontal groove (thumb)	Low level of basic life force
Unusually large or asymmetrical moons	High blood pressure
One or more moons missing	Imbalance in the nervous system Anemia Vitamin A deficiency Protein deficiency
Moons obscured, hard to see	Stroke Gastrointestinal disease Ulcer Asthma Acute pneumonia Gout
Separated from bed	Thyroid disorder Local infection
Pitted (like hammered brass)	Tendency toward hair loss
Pitted red-brown spots, with frayed and split ends	Psoriasis Need for vitamin C, folic acid, and protein
Beaded (bumps on surface)	Rheumatoid arthritis
Consistency	
Brittle	Iron deficiency Thyroid problems Impaired kidney function Circulatory problems
Brittle, soft, shiny, without moon	Overactive thyroid
Chip, peel, crack, break easily	General nutritional deficiency Insufficient hydrochloric acid Insufficient protein Insufficient minerals Vitamins A and D deficiency Thyroid problems Iron deficiency Calcium deficiency

Nail Signals	Potential Message (any or all may apply)
Consistency	
Thick	Circulatory problems Thyroid disease
Thinning	Lichen planus (itchy skin disorder)

Information Sources

Chinese Medical Palmistry, by Xiaofan Zong and Gary Liscum (Boulder, CO: Blue Poppy Press, 1995).

Healthy Healing, by Linda Rector-Page (Sacramento, CA: Spilman, 1990).

Prescription for Nutritional Healing, by James F. Balch and Phyllis A. Balch (Garden City Park, NY: Avery, 1997).

TONGUE OBSERVATIONS

Walk to the nearest mirror and stick out your tongue. Imagine that it has a tic-tac-toe grid drawn on it. According to the doctors and scientists who have studied these things, various internal organs affect the condition of the tongue, with each of these organs having a zone where its activities, or lack thereof, are reflected. Each of the nine boxes of the tic-tac-toe grid on your tongue thus corresponds to a key organ in your body.

Deepest into the mouth, at what is called the base of the tongue, the back row of boxes, from left to right (as you're looking at your tongue in the mirror), correspond to (L) left kidney, (M) large and small intestine, and (R) right kidney. The next row of boxes forward correspond to (L) spleen, (M) pancreas–duodenum–stomach, and (R) liver. The final row, at the front of the tongue, represent (L) left lung, (M) heart, and (R) right lung.

So here's the geography of your tongue:

Left kidney	Large and small intestine	Right kidney
Spleen	Pancreas, duodenum, and stomach	Liver
Left lung	Heart	Right lung

Again, the doctors and scientists who study these things tell us that the coloration, coating, and contour (or markings) of the overall tongue, and in particular in these nine individual areas, can tell a great deal about what's going on inside the body.

FROM THE SCIENCE OF ACUPUNCTURE

Professionals trained in the science of acupuncture are the most likely of all to make observations of the tongue when seeking to determine the health, or lack thereof, of the internal organs. From that arena come the following thoughts:

- Branches from the meridians of the kidney, heart, liver, spleen, lung, and stomach go through the tongue.

- The tip of the tongue reflects heart energy.

- The healthy tongue is:

    Full, but not thick

    Pink or pale red

    Thin, glistening, clear coat

    A little surface texture

- The color reflects the state of the blood and nourishing energy.

    Pale: deficient blood

    Red: heat pathology

- The shape reflects the state of the blood and nourishing energy.

    Thin or narrow reflects deficiency of blood

    Pale/swollen reflects spleen deficiency resulting in fluid retention

    Red/full reflects excess heat condition

- The degree of moisture reflects the condition of the body's fluids.

    Moist means fluids are not being transported well and are collecting in the body.

    Dry means a heat condition.

- The coating reflects the efficiency of the digestion, absorption, assimilation, and distribution functions of the stomach and spleen.

    White/thin coating is normal.

    Thicker white means slow digestion.

    Thick, in general, suggests a pathogenic process in the organs.

    Yellow reflects a heat problem.

(Coatings can be mixed, yellow in some zones and white in others, thick and thin, and mingled with raw or eroded surfaces. These represent multiple pathological processes at play in the same body.)

FROM OTHER HEALTH CARE APPROACHES

A search through the hundreds of books on nutrition and natural health care in my personal library revealed many similar thoughts about the appearance of the tongue and conditions it may indicate.

Color	Condition
Pink	Healthy
Dry, red tip	Heart problems
Black; bald spots on tongue; deep fissures (trenches)	Vitamin B3 deficiency
Reddened and/or smooth	Vitamin B6 (pyridoxine) deficiency
Cherry red or reddish-blue	Vitamin B2 deficiency
Red or inflamed	Malabsorption
Coating	
White	Systemic yeast infection
Contour	
Swollen	Food allergy
Inflamed or swollen	Vitamin B2 (riboflavin) deficiency Vitamin B12 (cobalamin) deficiency
Inflammation and/or soreness	Folic acid deficiency Iron deficiency
Geographic tongue (trenches)	Zinc deficiency
Geographic tongue and/or bald spots on tongue	Malabsorption

Are you still looking in that mirror? That's your best help available when it comes to tongue observations. You. Keep an eye on that tongue. Learn to read it well and regularly. When you brush your teeth, don't forget to brush your tongue; it will make it easier to distinguish discoloration and markings caused by internal problems as opposed to food particles.

Like many other forms of observation, tongue observation won't give you all the information you're seeking. But it is one more tool to put in your toolbox as you're learning how to read and take care of your body. As your health improves, expect that the overall condition of your tongue will, too.

URINE AND SALIVA pH TESTING

MOST AMERICANS ARE ACIDIC, primarily because of the standard American diet. All animal products, with the exception of butter, burn to acid ash as a result of the digestive process. Most cooked and otherwise processed foods do the same. While various parts of the body need to be more acidic than others, the health of the overall system depends on its being slightly alkaline. Cancer thrives in an acid environment.

What follows is information gleaned from the first book I was required to read as part of my training in naturopathy, *Your Health . . . Your Choice.* It is the single most important and comprehensive book I've read concerning pH testing and is available in the health section of most bookstores.

Here are important things to know about testing acid/alkaline balance:

The Paper

- Use paper that is calibrated in two-tenths increments.

- Paper registering between 5.5 and 8.0 is adequate, although the pH scale actually goes from 0 (total acid) to 14 (total alkaline).

- The pH Scale:

Total	Very	Moderate	Slight	Neutral	Slight	Moderate	Very	Total
0	1 2	3 4	5 6	7	8 9	10 11	12 13	14

- There is a tenfold change in intensity between each pH unit; for example, a reading of 5.0 is ten times more acid than 6.0.

- We make such paper available through Health*Quarters* Ministries.

The Urine pH

- MESSAGE: The first urine in the morning tells how your body handled the food you ate last night. It is a barometer of what's going on in the body and how drastically it may be adapting its various functions.

- BASELINE: Establish a baseline by checking the urine in the morning following a typical evening meal.

- TEST: Eat only acid ash–producing foods for the evening meal. You're looking for a pH between 5.5 and 5.8 the next morning. This is a sign that your body still has an adequate supply of neutralizing minerals (primarily organic sodium). When organic sodium is present in adequate amounts, urine pH registers as an acid after you have eaten acid foods. If you don't have enough reserve sodium, your urine pH will register 5.8 or above after a predominantly acid ash meal—a sign that the body is utilizing an emergency backup system to manufacture highly alkalinizing ammonia (pH 9.25) to neutralize acids. This is a sure sign that the body's alkaline reserve is depleted and resistance to disease is faltering.

- TARGET: If your urine pH is high after this test, it will begin to fall if you add meals to your menu that are alkalinizing (raw fruits and veggies). This may sound like the exact opposite of what you're hoping to achieve, but hang in there. As you continue to eat a primarily raw foods diet of fruits and veggies, your pH will eventually bottom out at about 5.5 and then begin climbing again. That's the goal—alkaline urine from eating alkaline foods. When you begin an 80/20 diet (80 percent raw fruits and veggies plus 20 percent cooked grains and veggies) you will be getting better as your urine pH drops, and getting healthy as it comes back up to toward 6.4 and 7.0.

The Saliva pH

- MESSAGE: The pH of saliva is representative of pH levels of most of your body fluids. The benchmark of 6.8 or above is ideal, whereas 6.2 is normal in the United States because of our acid-producing diet based on animal products and cooked or otherwise processed foods.

- BASELINE: Establish a baseline. Before eating, spit into a spoon, then dip paper. Check every two or three weeks after changing to 80/20 diet. Your pH should gradually go up toward increased alkalinity. It changes slowly.

- TEST: The most significant use of the saliva test is to see whether or not there is a dramatic change in the pH reading before and after a meal. Check saliva before you eat, then again about four minutes after you eat.

    Another approach is the lemon test. Lemon juice provides the physiological stimulus of a mini-meal. Check your saliva pH after having had nothing to eat for two hours or more. Just handling a lemon can send your saliva pH skyrocketing, so take this reading before picking it up. Squeeze a teaspoonful of juice into a spoon or glass of water. After consuming, wait two minutes before checking saliva pH.

    The acid in the lemon juice makes your mouth acidic. The mouth, however, is normally an alkaline environment. A major enzyme found in saliva, called amylase, is ineffective under acid conditions, so the body will work hard to counteract the acidity from the lemon juice. It does so by flooding the mouth with alkalinizing saliva. When you do the lemon test, you're looking to see if the pH goes up after you take some of the lemon.

- TARGET:

    If before a meal you're at 6.8, and afterward it jumps to 8.0 or higher, that's ideal.

    If before you're at 6.2, and afterward it rises higher, that's still good. It shows that you still have alkalinizing mineral reserves available.

    If you're at 5.5, but it does go up after eating, that's acceptable—not ideal, not good, but acceptable. It's an indication that, although you're low, you do still have some supply of alkalinizing minerals in your body.

If before the meal you're between 5.5 and 5.8 on the pH scale, and after eating there is no change, that's a sign that you need to get to work immediately to alkalinize your system. Your body is extremely acid, with inadequate mineral reserves available.

Finally, no matter what your pH was before a meal, if it goes down afterward that's an indication that your body chemistry, and thus pH reading, is being skewed by the impact of emotions that affect physiology. Some emotional detoxing would seem in order.

THE POINT

The whole point of pH testing is to see if your body has enough mineral reserves to continue to function properly. When those reserves wane, various sorts of disease processes can, and will, set in. Your body works continually to keep your blood pH at a consistent 7.4. If it drops to 7.2, you will die—it's that specific. The natural metabolic processes that body cells go through to generate energy result in acid waste by-products. This acid load the body must deal with is compounded when we feed ourselves a constant supply of acid. The body must draw heavily on mineral reserves to help keep the blood alkalinized, thus depleting its supply. As reserves dwindle, the body will begin to take calcium (an alkalinizing mineral) from bones. Osteoporosis, a weakening of bone structure, develops. Arthritis and kidney problems are not far behind, because of free-floating calcium the body must get rid of. The list of potential health problems could go on and on.

Bottom line: Good health is built upon a diet of alkalizing foods—raw fruits and vegetables. If you have trouble digesting them, try lightly steaming them along with taking enzyme supplements and hydrochloric acid. Gradually move toward more and more raw produce.

FURTHER READING

Your Health . . . Your Choice, by M. Ted Morter (Hollywood, FL: Lifetime Books, 1995).

STOOL OBSERVATIONS

The Four F's of Feces

WE HAD A FELLOW come to our Lodge a while back who admitted that he'd never bothered to turn around and see what he'd created after using the bathroom stool. What a shame. A great deal of information can be gleaned from one's bowel movements. Perhaps had he looked, he would have discovered clues of poor elimination that played a role in his eventual development of colon cancer.

By the time our friend left our Lodge, he'd not only learned to look, but he knew what to look for. You don't need a Ph.D. in "poopology" to be an expert.

ARE THEY FOUL?

Do your bowel movements stink? Contrary to popular belief, the stuff that comes out of us doesn't have to have the odoriferous power to remove paint. If what you leave in the stool is accompanied by an unpleasant odor, it's probably because food is rotting, putrefying, and fermenting in your digestive tract. More often than not this is due to one of two reasons:

1. Animal protein in the diet (the design of our intestinal tract makes for inefficient digestion of meat)

2. A lack of "friendly bacteria" in the intestines

The human intestinal tract (small and large intestines combined) contains as much as four and a half pounds of bacteria (living organisms). Some of these are "good guys," helping to promote health. Some are "bad guys"— *E. coli,* yeasts, molds, and fungi—that produce toxic substances, wound tissues, and can lead to any number of disease processes.

In *The Colon Health Handbook,* nutritionist Robert Gray points out that *E. coli* and related bad-guy bacteria in the human intestinal tract "produce a substance known as ethionine, which has been shown to cause cancer in laboratory animals."[1]

In a healthy intestinal tract, the good guys far outnumber the bad guys. Studies show the healthy balance to be at least 85 percent friendly with 15 percent or less bad-guy bacteria. The "friendlies" help to digest food by producing digestive enzymes and to manufacture certain vitamins vital to our health, particularly B1, B2, B6, biotin, and folic acid. They also serve to keep the bad guys in check.

Introduction of antibiotics, steroids, birth control pills, or any number of other drugs or chemicals that tend to be part of the modern American lifestyle can swing the balance of power to the "dark side." Typically, in most Americans' intestinal tracts, 85 percent of the bacteria are of the food-rotting, disease-producing type. When this happens, not only is food poorly digested, leading to gas, fermentation, and smelly bowel movements, but the walls of the intestinal tract can become wounded and porous due to the activity of the "unfriendlies." Toxic wastes are then reabsorbed back into the bloodstream through the wounds in the colon wall and delivered to every cell in the body. This process is called autointoxication. The body is poisoning itself because of reabsorption of its own waste products.

No doubt you're beginning to see how vitally important good flora are to the health of your intestinal tract, which in turn is important to the health of your entire body. Indeed, the British Medical Society has declared that "death begins in the colon."

What kind of flora to add? Good question. If you were to walk into any health food store in the country, you'd probably find several shelves of products displayed under the sign "Flora" or, the more fancy term, "Probiotics." More often than not they're kept in a refrigeration display case. If

---

Just remember "the four F's of feces":

• Are they foul?
• Are they frequent?
• Are they formed?
• Are they floating?

Frähm's Principle of Colon Health

If your feces are foul, add some flora!

you ask an employee for assistance in finding their flora display, he or she will probably say, "You're looking for acidophilus." Actually, *acidophilus* is the name given to one of several different kinds of beneficial bacteria, but it has come to denote the entire family of good-for-you flora.

At Health*Quarters* Ministries we've tried different brands and blends with our Lodge guests and supplement customers. The one we like best is a product called PB8. It contains not just one but eight different strains of friendly bacteria. It's produced in such a way as to be stable at room temperature—in other words, it doesn't need refrigeration. And it has the highest potency available on the market. Besides all that, it comes in specially coated capsules that keep the bacteria from being destroyed by digestive juices in the stomach before they can reach the intestines.

What's that, you're asking? Won't eating yogurt give me the acidophilus my body needs? Probably not. First of all, acidophilus cultures are destroyed when mixed with the fruits so often used to flavor yogurts. Even in plain yogurts, the level of good bacteria decreases rapidly in just a few days' time.

If you're buying plain yogurt from a store, it's a good bet those products were manufactured weeks earlier. Even if some of the bacteria linger, they're destroyed by the gastric juices in the stomach before reaching the intestinal tract, where they're most needed. Again, if your feces are foul (and/or you have smelly gas), add some flora. You might want to consider PB8.

Note: Eating meat sets up conditions in the bowel that are conducive to putrefaction and fermentation because of the long time meat requires to travel through the human digestive tract. For health reasons, and especially if you're fighting a disease process like cancer, removing meat from your daily diet would be a prudent move. Once you're out of the proverbial "woods" healthwise, your body may be better able to handle the challenge of dealing with meat.

ARE THEY FREQUENT?

Nutritionists, naturopaths, and nutritionally minded doctors will tell you that it's healthy to have at least two to three bowel movements a day. Any backup of wastes in the colon can lead to reabsorption of toxins into the bloodstream—considered by many the forerunner of degenerative disease.

On the other hand, the National Cancer Institute says that it's within "normal" range for the average American to have as few as three bowel movements a week.[2] Obviously, what's "normal" is not always what's healthy.

So what's the answer to maintaining a healthy bowel function? Fiber! Fiber is to your intestinal tract what a broom and mop are to a kitchen floor. It sweeps up debris and absorbs toxins, moving them toward removal. It also absorbs water, creating bulky stools and thus helping to tone the bowel muscle by giving it something to push against.

It's of interest to note that no dietary fiber exists in any animal products (meat of all kinds and dairy). Since animal products are the focus of the standard American diet (S.A.D.), it's "normal" for the average American to have a weak, flabby intestinal tract that is slow and clogged up.

Fiber comes from plants. Even the National Cancer Institute, not known for its emphasis on nutrition in fighting disease, is doing all it can to inform and encourage the American public to eat five to nine helpings of fruits and vegetables every day. They are an excellent source of dietary fiber.

Again, an early warning sign that you may be setting up conditions for the advent of a disease process in your body is the slowing down of your bowel. Are you getting your five to nine servings of fruit and vegetables daily? If not, you'd do well to add some supplemental fiber to your diet. Psyllium husks and psyllium husk powders are most commonly used for this purpose.

At Health*Quarters* we're big fans of a product called Perfect 7. It's a unique blend of psyllium seeds and husks with friendly flora, bentonite, alfalfa leaf, cascara sagrada bark, rose hips, buckthorn bark, capsicum, garlic, and goldenseal.

Note: Always drink lots of water when taking fiber. Your minimum daily water needs are determined by dividing your body weight in half. Consider this in ounces. For example, a 200-pound man needs to drink 100 ounces a day as a bare minimum. Divide this by 8 and you get the total number of 8-ounce glasses. When adding fiber to your diet, it's a good idea to exceed minimum water requirements. Keep that fiber moving!

In addition, consider eliminating salt and dairy from your diet. Both tend to be constipating. Dairy is mucus-forming, clogging up the bowel. Salt in the diet makes the blood salty. This draws water into the bloodstream from the intestines where that fluid was meant to keep stools soft. The result is dry, hard-to-pass fecal matter.

Frähm's Principle of Colon Health

If your feces aren't frequent, add fiber!

ARE THEY FORMED?

It is a commonly held notion within nutrition circles that a perfectly healthy bowel movement is about two feet long (the length extending from the top of the descending part of the colon on the left side of your body all the way down to your anus) and has the approximate diameter of a half dollar.

Ah, perfection—who can attain it? Several things will help you progress toward movements of this magnitude. The importance of adding flora and fiber to your diet has already been discussed. To these, add digestive help in the form of supplemental hydrochloric acid (HCl). A poorly formed stool is often a sign that food is not being well digested. This is not good.

"Proper digestion," write Michael Murray, N.D., and Joseph Pizzorno, N.D., authors of the *Encyclopedia of Natural Medicine,* "is a requirement for optimum health. Incomplete or disordered digestion can be a major contributor to the development of many diseases."[3]

When digestion is not good, our bodies don't break down and assimilate the nutrients in foods, no matter how good their quality. Incompletely digested food particles, particularly proteins, can also be inappropriately absorbed into the bloodstream. This leads to the advent of food allergies, a general weakening of immune power, and the potential onset of various disease processes.

Hydrochloric acid is the digestive fluid in the stomach essential for beginning the process of breaking down foods, particularly proteins. As it does its job, it signals the pancreas to send forth a supply of the digestive enzymes it produces into the small intestine, where digestion and absorption continue.

The reason it's important to supplement your diet with hydrochloric acid (or at least check yourself to see if you're needing it) is that about the time we turn 30 years of age, we tend to produce less and less. Studies indicate that as many as 9 out of every 10 Americans over the age of 30 have low stomach acidity. Without sufficient HCL, food is not well digested, the pancreas never gets the signal to flood the small intestine with enzymes, and all kinds of problems develop.

According to Murray and Pizzorno, the following are common when stomach acidity is low:[4]

Symptoms

Bloating, belching, burning, and flatulence immediately after meals

A sense of fullness after eating

Indigestion, diarrhea, or constipation

Multiple food allergies

Nausea after taking supplements

Itching around the rectum

Signs

Weak, peeling, and cracked fingernails

Dilated blood vessels in the cheeks and nose (in nonalcoholics)

Acne

Iron deficiency

Chronic intestinal parasites or abnormal flora

Undigested food in stool

Chronic candida infections

Upper digestive tract gassiness

Associated Disease Processes

Addison's disease

Asthma

Cancer (my addition, based on what I've studied and seen— why they didn't include this in their list, I don't know)

Celiac disease

Chronic autoimmune disorders

Chronic hives

Diabetes mellitus

Eczema

Gallbladder disease

Graves' disease

Hepatitis

Hyper- and hypothyroidism

Lupus erythematosus

Myasthenia gravis

Osteoporosis

Pernicious anemia

Psoriasis

Rheumatoid arthritis

Rosacea

Sjögren's syndrome

Thyrotoxicosis

Vitiligo

**Frähm's Principle
of Colon Health**

If your feces aren't
formed, add hydrochloric
acid (HCl) and enzymes.
Of course, don't leave
out the flora and fiber
either!

It's interesting to take note of all the commercials shown on TV suggesting antacid products, when in most cases just the opposite is required. Most of us (9 out of 10) need more acid in our stomachs, not less. A capsule or two of supplemental hydrochloric acid or a little lemon juice in water (a natural form of HCl) would in most cases do what the body needs done. Even a teaspoon of vinegar will often add the acid to the digestive process that the stomach is missing. The reason antacids often seem to bring temporary relief is that they tell the stomach to simply quit trying and just push the stuff off into the intestinal tract.

As important as hydrochloric acid is, so are enzymes. Your pancreas manufactures lipases, which digest fat, proteases, which digest protein, and amylases, which digest starches. If and when the pancreas gets the signal from the HCl that food is in the stomach and headed for the small intestines, it will gladly send forth a supply. But as we've seen, this signal does not always come. In some cases the signal comes, but the pancreas is simply unable, for whatever reasons, to adequately respond.

It appears highly beneficial, therefore, since HCl and enzymes work together as the dynamic duo of digestion, to supplement the diet with both.

What kind should you use?

There are many, many different brands and product formulas on the market that might work for you. Here at HQM we use a product called Food Enzymes from Nature's Sunshine Products that combines HCl with several different kinds of digestive enzymes, adding to the mix some important cofactors that enhance the effectiveness of both. (Either follow directions for the amount on the bottle or use your newly acquired skill at muscle response testing—see chapter 28—to see how many your system needs.)

DO THEY FLOAT?

Last but not least, you want feces that float. You don't want the kind that submarine to the bottom of the toilet like a rock. It's "floaters" you're after, not "sinkers."

I know that sounds funny and odd, but sinkers are a sign that your bowel movements are hard and compact. A healthy stool is one that is loosely formed, floats, and breaks up into smaller pieces when flushed. When your bowel movements sink, something's missing in your diet. That something, more often than not, is either fiber, essential fatty acids, or both.

We've already discussed the necessity of fiber. Let's take a closer look at the need for essential fatty acids (EFAs).

Not all fats are destructive to one's health. Whereas saturated fats found in meat and dairy products tend to clog arteries and lead to circulatory problems and other diseases (as do "trans" fatty acids, found in margarine), there are certain fats that our bodies need in order to carry on several vital functions. These fats are called essential fatty acids—"essential" referring to the fact that our bodies don't produce them, so they must come from our diet. (Anything that the human body requires to maintain health but doesn't naturally make is referred to as an essential nutrient.)

There are two classes of EFAs: Omega-3 and Omega-6. Both are important in the maintenance of healthy cells. Flaxseed oil, a product we use here at HQM, is the richest vegetable source of Omega-3 fatty acids (52 percent) and also provides a good supply of Omega-6 (20 percent).

Because it is so rich in these vital nutrients, flaxseed oil is a building block for healthy cells and membranes; it has been shown to be especially useful in the treatment of degenerative diseases. Studies have shown that it can actually help cancerous cells change back into healthy ones.

SUMMARY

Turn around. Take a look. Evaluate. You want frequent bowel movements that are well formed, float, and don't smell bad.

Frähm's Principles of Colon Health

- If your feces are foul, add some flora!
- If your feces aren't frequent, add fiber!
- If your feces aren't formed, add hydrochloric acid (HCl) and enzymes. Of course, don't leave out the flora and fiber either!
- If your feces don't float, add flaxseed oil and fiber!

PART 6

A HERO'S

TRAITS

36

CHARACTERISTICS
OF THOSE WHO
DO WELL

YOU MADE IT FAR. You examined the "rocks" that tend to weigh heavily against the average body's ability to maintain health. You learned important tools for cleaning out and strengthening your system. You got some ideas about how to keep track of how your body is responding to the help you're giving.

It's time for me to share with you the characteristics of people who have done well on self-help, self-directed programs of health recovery like this. These observations have been made as I've watched people go through the Lodge program and as I've read or heard health recovery stories from those who have read our books and contacted Health*Quarters* Ministries.

LIVE MESSAGES

A few years back a woman called the Health*Quarters* office saying that she'd like to tell us her story. One day she had found a lump in her breast. Naturally concerned, she wasted no time making tracks for her friendly doctor's office. A biopsy revealed the lump to be cancerous. Mastectomy was offered as her only option. Aware of no other ways in which to deal with this condition, she agreed to the surgery.

Characteristic to Cultivate

Sending your body "thumbs up" signals—live messages

Following up the mastectomy, she was told in no uncertain terms that it was necessary for her to undergo "preventive" chemotherapy. Preventive chemotherapy? Now that the tumor had been removed and the overall cancer load reduced, why not work to revive and stimulate the immune system that allowed the tumor to develop in the first place—get her immune system to clean up leftover cancer cells? What were her doctors thinking?

Yes, I know. But that's not the way docs think who have been trained in allopathic ("invade and stop") medicine. Their attention and tools are aimed at attacking symptoms, rather than rebuilding and stimulating the body's healing powers. And so, she agreed to it. Who wouldn't? When such a thing is presented to us as the only "right" thing to do, who among us can argue?

The chemo made her sick, but after it was over and her hair grew back, all seemed right in the world once again. She was told to go enjoy the rest of her life. This had been her brush with the disease. Time now to get on with her life.

A year came and went. All seemed fine. And it was fine . . . all the way up until that day when she found a lump in the other breast. This, too, turned out to be cancer. Discouragement threatened to swallow her whole. But, true to her nature, and to her sense of being in God's hands, she wouldn't let it.

"I'm determined to beat this thing," she told her doctors.

Chemo was once again offered. This time she refused.

Tamoxifen was next—a relative newcomer to the allopathic cancer-fighting team. It would help to block estrogens from feeding her tumor. She gave it a try. In her case—not in every case, but in her case—it made her cancer grow.

Taxol followed. It, too, was a relative newcomer to the allopathic approach to cancer. And although it was a chemotherapeutic agent, the kind of thing she'd told her doctors she didn't want to do again, she gave it a shot.

In her case—not in every case, but in her case—Taxol made her quit breathing. She was having an "anaphylactic" reaction to the stuff. Immediate hospitalization was required to purge her system.

"There's one last hope for you," her doctors said. "A bone marrow transplant."

After much discussion and prayer with her family, it was decided that she'd do it. She'd leave her small town and head to a special hospital far away from home where they were renowned in such matters. The entire family went to be supportive.

Upon arrival, she was examined by the doctor who was to be her attending physician during her stay. As he finished and stepped back to review his notes, he scratched his head and told her that the tumor in her breast was too large for a bone marrow transplant to be of any help.

The "thunk" that could be heard was her heart hitting bottom.

Once again discouragement stood at the door, ready to pounce and devour. Once again, she refused. Turning to her family she simply said, "I'm no closer to death today than I was yesterday. Let's go home and find a way to beat this stuff."

That next Sunday found them sitting in church, back home. Someone who had heard news of their plight handed them a book. It just happened to be the one that my wife and I had written, *A Cancer Battle Plan*.

"I devoured the book," she said. "In the town here I found a chiropractor who was also trained in nutrition. He helped me with juice fasting, and my diet and supplements. And in a nearby town I discovered a woman who helped me learn the fine art of water and coffee enemas."

Shortly after launching herself in this direction, she paid her doctor a visit. "Well," he said, after hearing about what she was trying, "you'd better have a plan B."

"Plan B! I've tried all your plan As! You figure out a plan B!" And off she went.

"That was about a year ago," she said as she eagerly told us her story that day on the phone. "I just wanted to call to thank you for writing that book. I worked hard at detoxifying my body and renewing its healing power, and it was my body that took care of the disease. Today I am cancer free."

The thing we learned from that lady, and from so many others who have done well in winning back their health from the clutches of cancer, is the importance of giving our bodies "thumbs up" signals—or in other words, "live messages."

At every turn this woman faced the possibility of being overwhelmed by discouragement and frustration. At any point, and especially when told that the bone marrow transplant was not possible, she could have thrown in the towel—given up.

When a person begins to tell his or her body that it's doomed, it will be. There truly is a strong mind/body link. What you think will impact your health. If you start sending death messages to your body, it will indeed die.

LIVING PURPOSEFULLY

I was for a number of years a career consultant. I enjoyed helping people clarify their sense of purpose, then pursue it with passion. Within this setting I learned that if a man retires from his work at age 65 with no plan as to what to accomplish with the rest of his years, he tends to live an average of another 13½ months. Now that is a waste. Lack of purpose can be deadly. On the other hand, pursuing one's sense of purpose is life giving.

Way back when my wife first found out that she was battling cancer, one of the first things we did was to start a business for her. She was a gifted artist, with an eye for color and design. She'd always loved to decorate and redecorate our own home, and she had a deep and abiding passion to help bring beauty into the homes and lives of others.

Her new business, helping to fulfill her sense of purpose, was a key part of her cancer battle plan. It helped her get out of bed in the morning, and it pulled her forward into life. Eventually it gave way to yet another purpose, that of giving birth to Health*Quarters* Ministries. Hers was a "purpose-filled" life. I'm convinced that this was a key part of why she did so well against such overwhelming odds.

In her, and in so many others, I've seen that people who do well on a self-directed journey toward renewed health are people who have a purpose for living—a sense of what they feel called to contribute to this world. More than just to live to see a child married or to experience one more Christmas or to take some long-desired trip, they've gotten in touch with what they believe to be the reason why God has them here on this earth— the contribution He wants them to make.

There's nothing like cancer to help a person get in touch with what's really important, why he or she is really here. Here are some questions that can help the clarification process. Pick one or two that spark a response and write out your thoughts.

- What need do I see that I'd like to be part of meeting?
- What wrong do I see that I'd like to address?
- What opportunity do I see that I'd like to make the most of?
- What cause would I like to serve?

Characteristic to Cultivate

Seeking to clarify and live out a sense of purpose for your life

- What contribution could I make to this world to make it a better place?

- What do I want written about me when I'm gone?

- If time, money, and the opinion of others were of no importance, what would I be doing with my life?

DISCIPLINED CHANGE

In your cancer battle plan this can be the hardest. People who do well, people who have succeeded at winning back their health in the face of even the worst of odds, are people who have successfully cultivated the ability to make disciplined change. The things we choose to expose ourselves to and the diets we feed our bodies are the key contributors to the fact that one out of every two Americans will develop cancer. Cancer demands change. Disciplined change. And to areas of our lives where we tend to resist change the most.

Two ladies came to our Lodge a while back. I'll call them Jane and Mary. Both had breast cancer.

Jane decided that once she got back home she'd have no time to work on her health. She and her husband ran a business that in reality ran them. They chose not to make changes. Within six months, Jane ran out of time.

Mary, on the other hand, along with her husband, decided that wholesale changes would be made. Nothing would stand in the way of their efforts to regain her health. Every aspect of their lifestyle was put up for inspection. Hard choices were made. Changes were enforced. Today Mary is cancer free and doing well.

From these two and hundreds more like them, I've seen that people who tend to do well at winning back their health are those who are willing to make whatever changes are necessary. And in the process they discipline themselves to stick with it. Resisting change, only to end up out of time, is your proverbial "bummer."

PARTNERSHIP

People who do well at winning back their health are people who have formed partnerships with others who are "on fire" for what it takes. Without such partnership, the flame of change tends to die out quickly. Some

Characteristic to Cultivate

Searching after partnership like your life depends on it; it just might

may be able to enjoy the "fire" that a supportive spouse can provide. Life, however, isn't always the way we wish. When it comes to diet changes, a mate can sometimes act more like a bucket of cold water. That doesn't make your mate bad or evil—just not yet ready to catch fire.

In my experience, husbands are more often like this than wives. It's often hard to convince a man to make changes to his diet and lifestyle unless he comes face to face with a health crisis of his own.

Anyhow, the bottom line is that those who tend to be successful at winning back their health are people who have either found or created partnership to help keep them going in the things they need to do.

Here are a couple of examples of how to ignite interest in others.

Start a nutrition and natural health support group.
Anne and I began such a group shortly after her original success against cancer. We decided to gather our friends and teach them all we'd learned about how to feed and take care of our bodies. Four friends responded to our invitation.

After our second meeting, frustrated with our own ignorance and the time it took to prepare to teach others, we hit on a "gold mine" of an idea. From that point on, each bimonthly meeting in our home featured a guest speaker—a professional from the community who had some service to offer within the realm of nutrition and/or natural health.

We heard from nutritionists, massage therapists, biologically trained dentists, a medical doctor who did chelation therapy, naturopathic and homeopathic doctors, chiropractors, a colonic therapist, an organic gardener, a nutritional bread maker, a stretching expert, an exercise specialist, and more.

Within a short time word had spread. Sixty people were showing up twice a month in our living room. Anne and I would move the furniture and rent a trunkload of "skinny butt" chairs, and twice a month we'd all get to hear what a different health-related professional had to say. We'd get free teaching, and they'd get an opportunity to tell potential clients what they had to offer.

Eventually the whole thing got so incredibly popular that we had to ask our church if we could meet in the church basement. At one point the ranks of those who were attending our support group had swollen to 120—30 times the number we'd begun with!

You, too, can create "fire" like this. You don't need to be a teacher—

just a facilitator. Find a place to meet. A home is a great location—at least until the crowd gets too big. Locate various professionals in your community whom you'd like to hear and invite them to speak to your group. Let all your friends know they can come hear and get to know "this or that" doctor or health-related professional without having to pay for an appointment.

Ask each person who comes to chip in a couple of bucks in order to present your speaker with an honorarium for his or her time and presentation. This will go a long way toward ensuring a repeat performance down the road.

Start a co-op.
A while back one of the ladies who went through our Lodge program got an idea that perhaps getting some of her neighborhood friends interested in healthy eating would help her to stay focused that way herself.

As she began to kick around ideas, she ran across a company that was willing to deliver organic produce to her garage twice a month if she was able to make it worth their time by placing a big enough order. That was just the spark she needed to create "fire." Over the next few days she contacted and convinced 30 of her neighbor ladies to place orders with her on a monthly basis.

Not only did this co-op idea help to keep her eating the way she knew she should, but she was able to make enough money from it to cover the cost of her own produce. She simply added a surcharge of 5 percent to each neighbor's order. It was, after all, her idea and her garage.

The fringe benefit to the whole thing, of course, was the platform of common interest that this co-op established among these 30 neighborhood households. Lives were opened up to each other like never before, and all because of one lady's need and willingness to try to create partnership.

Bottom line, you're going to need the help and encouragement of like-minded people as you make your way toward renewed health. If you're not one to want to try to create something, look for a nutrition/natural health support group that's already started.

LITTLE THINGS

I have noted over the years that people who seem to do the best at winning back their health are those who take a hard look at every area of their lives.

Characteristic to Cultivate

Paying attention to even the little things

Characteristic to Cultivate

Finding peace with and through the God of the Bible

They leave no "rock" unturned. A lot of little stresses on your body, just like a lot of little rocks in a car's trunk, make for a heavy load.

Rhonda came to our Lodge fresh from a diagnosis of breast cancer and full of the fear that such news brings. "I'm here to change my whole life," she said. Blessed by strong support from her husband, she did just that. Everything from her diet to the kind of toothpaste she used to the way she handled her anger was evaluated. Wholesale changes were implemented.

Today Rhonda is not just surviving, she's thriving.

Remember, what seems at first a little thing may actually turn out to be a much bigger stress on your body than you ever thought.

Go back through chapters 3–8 and look at the "rocks" once again. What things have you maybe not paid enough attention to? Still drinking tap water? Haven't yet got yourself checked for parasites? Haven't yet seen a biologically trained dentist about your root canals? Haven't yet decided to practice forgiveness toward that ex of yours?

Those people who tend to do well do at first work on what appear to be the big "rocks" in their "trunks." That only makes sense. But they don't stop there. They echo Rhonda's sentiment, "I'm here to change my whole life."

PEACE WITH GOD

I have noted that people who tend to do well on a self-help journey toward renewing their health are people who have put their confidence in God.

There is a quality about these folks that I find in no others. They display a peace of mind about their situation—a relaxed confidence that regardless of their physical outcome, they are in the strong hands of a Father who cares. It's as if they know that there's more to life than is seen.

I note that such a relationship with God tends to lift the emotional load, allowing more energy to go toward physical healing. "A heart at peace," says the Bible, "gives life to the body" (Proverbs 14:30).

Think about it.

These, then, are the six characteristics I've seen in those who have done well using a cancer battle plan like that outlined in the pages of this book.

1. They send their bodies "thumbs up" or live messages.

2. They seek to clarify and live out a sense of direction and purpose for their lives.

3. They are willing to make disciplined changes.

4. They seek partnership that will help them stay true to their health goals.

5. They give attention to even the little things.

6. They trust the God of the Bible.

APPENDIX A:
HEALTH*QUARTERS*
MINISTRIES
RESOURCES

To Contact Us

955C Garden of the Gods Rd.
Colorado Springs, CO 80907
(719) 593-8694
(719) 531-7884 (FAX)
e-mail: HealthQuarters@juno.com
Website: www.healthquarters.org

To Place an Order

Throughout this book I've been telling you about things available through HQM. Here is how to place an order:

1. Have your credit card ready.
2. Give us a call at (719) 593-8694 (M–F, 8 A.M.–4 P.M. Mountain Time).
3. Or place an order on our Website: www.healthquarters.org

A review of things we make available:

- Key books and supplements
- Reverse osmosis water filtering systems
- Alpine air purification systems
- Champion juicers
- Health Resources List (a national listing of professionals who use nutrition and/or nontoxic therapies)
- Free monthly newsletter

For a full description of all that we carry, order a copy of our catalog.

The HealthQuarters Lodge Program

Concept: a "diet and lifestyle change center" aimed at helping fellow Christians learn how to be better stewards of their health so that they can more effectively accomplish all that God wants them to do in this life.

It's hard to serve when you're sick.

Program

- 11 days (leave on day 11)
- Body detoxification education and experience, including seven-day juice fast with colon/liver cleansings
- Personalized nutritional assessment by Dave Frähm
- Nutrition classes with Dave Frähm
- Personal health care products education
- "How to read your own body" education
- Health food store field trip
- Prayer sessions and devotionals
- Mild exercise and relaxation
- Therapeutic massage
- Health Resources List—a link to professional help back home
- One-year "Going Home" plan for diet and continuing body detox
- *Optional:* "Going Home" supplement package

Important Note: Our Lodge program does not include nursing care, drugs, or medications. We are not a hospital, clinic, treatment center, or hospice.

We do not label symptoms or illnesses, prescribe drugs, or treat disease. We are an education/resource center for lifestyle changes, led by Dave Frähm—nutritionist, naturopath, and educator. The design of our program has participants fully involved in hands-on application of what they're learning. If you are incapable of a self-administered program, we can suggest other facilities that would better meet your needs.

APPENDIX B:
QUESTIONS
AND ANSWERS

Where can I get a gauss meter?
   The Cutting Edge Catalog
   P.O. Box 5034
   New York, NY 11969
   (800) 497-9516
   (516) 287-3813 (NY metro area)
   (516) 287-3112 (FAX)
   e-mail: cutcat@cutcat.com
   Website: www.cutcat.com

   Their Cellsensor Meter is the cheapest of their gauss meters.

Where can I get "study at home" education in nutrition and natural health?
   Trinity School of Natural Health
   401 Kings Highway
   Winona Lake, IN 46590
   (800) 428-0408
   (219) 267-6111

What are your three favorite books in the field of natural health?

Alternative Medicine, by the Burton Goldberg Group (Tiburon, CA: Future Medicine, 1993).

Definitive Guide to Cancer, by W. John Diamond and W. Lee Cowden with Burton Goldberg (Tiburon, CA: Future Medicine, 1997).

Prescription for Nutritional Healing, by James F. Balch and Phyllis A. Balch (Garden City Park, NY: Avery, 1997).

All three are available from Health*Quarters* Ministries.

What kind of health insurance do you personally have?

I'm actually part of a nationwide group where we've agreed to share each others' medical costs. It's called the Christian Care Medi-Share Program and is a program of the Christian Care Ministry.

The cost for a family is *much* less than typical health insurance and comes with a corporate emphasis on healthy lifestyles, both physically and spiritually. At a certain level of claim, a catastrophic insurance policy does kick in.

The group's newsletter, *Helping One Another,* is sent out on a monthly basis, and it is loaded with information on nutrition and natural health.

Although this plan is not insurance, the group has set up special criteria to help determine who can join. Pre-existent cancer would exclude a person. If that's true of you, this may still be a great program for your other family members . . . and eventually for you, once you've been cancer free for a qualifying period of time.

If you're interested in exploring the possibility of becoming a member of Christian Care Medi-Share, contact:

Joe Foreman
Chartered Financial Consultant
5101 SW 34th St.
Topeka, KS 66614-3909
(800) 268-2514
foreman@we-communicate.com

Let him know that you've been referred by Dave Frähm.

NOTES

Chapter 1: Your Body Is the Hero
1. Psalm 139:13–14, *Living Bible* (Wheaton, IL: Tyndale House, 1971).

Chapter 3: Toxic Diet
1. John A. McDougall and Mary A. McDougall, *The McDougall Plan* (Piscataway, NJ: New Century, 1983), page 95.
2. Maureen Salaman, *Nutrition: The Cancer Answer* (Menlo Park, CA: Statford Publishing, 1984), pages 75, 76.
3. Julian Whitaker and June Roth, *Reversing Health Risks* (New York: Putnam, 1988), page 80.
4. Harvey Diamond and Marilyn Diamond, *Fit for Life* (New York: Warner Books, 1985), page 71.
5. JoAnn Rachor, *Of These You May Freely Eat* (Sunfield, MI: Family Health, 1986), page 83.
6. W. John Diamond and W. Lee Cowden with Burton Goldberg, *Definitive Guide to Cancer* (Tiburon, CA: Future Medicine, 1997), page 774.
7. Whitaker and Roth, page 84.
8. Diamond and Cowden with Goldberg, page 572.

9. Michael F. Jacobson, Lisa Y. Lefferts, and Anne Witte Garland, *Safe Food* (Los Angeles: Living Planet Press, 1991), page 48.

10. Ibid.

11. John Robbins, "Realities for the Nineties," in *Diet for a New America,* by John Robbins (Walpole, NH: Stillpoint, 1987).

12. Jacobson, Lefferts, and Garland, page 59.

13. Michael Murray and Joseph Pizzorno, *Encyclopedia of Natural Medicine* (Rocklin, CA: Prima, 1991), page 34.

14. Jacobson, Lefferts, and Garland, pages 150–170.

15. Ibid., page 163.

16. Joel Robbins, *Enzymes for Health* (cassette tape presentation), available from Vitality Unlimited, P.O. Box 322, Colonia, NJ 07067, 1-800-93-VITAL.

Chapter 4: Toxic Dentistry

1. Hal Huggins, "Results of the Coors Blood Chemistry Study on the Effects of Dental Mercury Amalgam Fillings and Recent Investigations into the Toxicity of Root Canals and Cavitations," *Townsend Letter for Doctors and Patients,* July 1997, page 84.

2. Hal Huggins, "Dental Toxins: Your Teeth May Be Making You Sick," *Alternative Medicine Digest,* May 1998, page 52.

3. Thomas Levy, "Teeth: The Root of Most Disease," *Extraordinary Science,* April/May/June 1994.

4. Ibid., page 50.

5. George E. Meinig, *Root Canal Cover-Up* (Ojai, CA: Bion, 1996), page 25.

6. Burton Goldberg Group, *Alternative Medicine* (Tiburon, CA: Future Medicine, 1993), page 87.

7. Ibid., page 86.

8. Ibid., page 94.

9. Julian Whitaker, "You Don't Need Fluoridated Water," *Health and Healing Newsletter,* September 1997, page 5.

10. Ibid., pages 4, 5.

11. Ibid., page 9.

12. Ibid.

13. Robert C. Olney, "Stop Fluoride Diseases," *Cancer Forum,* page 8.

14. W. John Diamond and W. Lee Cowden with Burton Goldberg, *Definitive Guide to Cancer* (Tiburon, CA: Future Medicine, 1997), pages 580–581.

15. Sherry Rogers, *Northeast Center for Environmental Medicine Health Letter,* July/August 1996 (Prestige Publishing, Syracuse, NY 13220, 1-800-846-6687).

Chapter 5: Toxic Emotions

1. Proverbs 4:30, *New International Version Study Bible* (Grand Rapids, MI: Zondervan, 1985), page 965.
2. W. John Diamond and W. Lee Cowden with Burton Goldberg, *Definitive Guide to Cancer* (Tiburon, CA: Future Medicine, 1997), page 140.

Chapter 6: Toxic Environment

1. Dan Fagan, "Are You at Risk from Sick Building Syndrome?" *Family Circle,* April 25, 1995, page 71.
2. James F. Balch, *The Super Anti-Oxidants* (New York: M. Evans, 1998), page 35.
3. Lily Giambarba Casura, "Rx for Winter Health: Breathe Green Air," *Townsend Letter for Doctors and Patients,* December 1997, page 68.
4. Environmental Health Foundation of Tucson, AZ, as quoted by Diane de Simone, "Air Raid," *Country Living's Healthy Living.*
5. B. C. Wolverton, *How to Grow Fresh Air: 50 Houseplants That Purify Your Home or Office* (New York: Penguin Books, 1996), page 13.
6. United States Environmental Protection Agency, *Residential Air-Cleaning Devices: A Summary of Available Information,* Washington, D.C., February 1990.
7. Casura, page 69.
8. Joseph D. Weissman, *Choose to Live* (New York: Penguin Books, 1988), page 46.
9. Elson M. Haas, *Staying Healthy with Nutrition* (Berkeley, CA: Celestial Arts, 1992), page 17.
10. Alan R. Gaby, "Research Review," *Nutrition and Healing,* November 1994, page 7.
11. Weissman, page 222.
12. W. John Diamond and W. Lee Cowden with Burton Goldberg, *Definitive Guide to Cancer* (Tiburon, CA: Future Medicine, 1997), page 580.
13. Weissman, page 62.
14. Andrew Weil, *8 Weeks to Optimum Health* (New York: Knopf, 1997), page 65.
15. Julian Whitaker, "Save Your Skin from the Sun," *Health and Healing,* July 1995, page 6.

16. Deborah Sarnoff, "Fun in the Sun," *Delicious,* April 1994, page 54.

17. Ross Anderson, "Are You Clear of Parasites?" page 2.

18. Ibid.

19. Sam Biser, *Rejuvenate Your Body by Eliminating Parasites,* A Special Report from Swanannoa Institute, 1990, pages 9, 10.

20. Ann Louise Gittleman, *Guess What Came to Dinner* (Garden City Park, NY: Avery, 1993), page 38.

21. Ibid., page 52.

22. Ellen Reeder, "Parasites: Uninvited Guests," brochure obtained from Bioclinics-Minneapolis, 7275 Washington Ave. S., Edna, MN 55439, (612) 996-0770.

Chapter 7: Toxic Lifestyle

1. Andrew Weil, *Natural Health, Natural Medicine* (Boston: Houghton Mifflin, 1990), pages 135, 136.

2. George Milowe, "Help Stop the Tobacco Epidemic," *Townsend Letter for Doctors and Patients,* August/September 1994, page 943.

3. Ibid., page 3.

4. Aileen Ludington and Hans Diehl, *Dynamic Living* (Hagerstown, MD: Review and Herald, 1995), page 37.

5. Dan Hurley, "Reasons to Quit Smoking Abound," *Gazette Telegraph* (Colorado Springs), January 3, 1995.

6. Daisy Chan, *Total Health,* vol. 20, no. 5, page 10.

7. James F. Balch, *The Super Anti-Oxidants* (New York: M. Evans, 1998), page 33.

8. Ibid.

9. Associated Press, "Smoking Mom's Babies 'Ex-Smokers'", *Gazette Telegraph (Colorado Springs),* March 20, 1997.

10. Stuart M. Berger, *How to Be Your Own Nutritionist* (New York: William Morrow, 1987), page 140.

11. Weil, page 133.

12. Associated Press, "Drinking during Pregnancy Raises Leukemia Risk for Baby, Study Shows," *Gazette Telegraph* (Colorado Springs), January 3, 1996.

13. Andrew Weil, *Spontaneous Healing* (New York: Fawcett Columbine, 1995), page 190.

14. Jeffrey Moss, "Sleep—The Great, Overlooked Antioxidant?" *Townsend Letter for Doctors and Patients,* January 1996, page 120.

15. Dean Ornish, *Eat More, Weigh Less* (New York: HarperPerennial, 1993), page 5.

Chapter 8: Toxic Medical Practices and Procedures

1. Sherry Rogers, *Northeast Center for Environmental Medicine Health Letter,* July/August 1996 (later known as *Total Health in Today's World*).

2. James F. Balch, *The Super Anti-Oxidants* (New York: M. Evans, 1998), page 27.

3. Sydney M. Wolfe, *Women's Health Alert* (New York: Addison-Wesley, 1991), page 25.

4. W. Lee Cowden, *Preventing and Reversing Cancer* (cassette tape series), Great Health, Richardson, TX, (972) 480–8909.

5. Ellen Hodgson Brown, "Studies Raise New Questions about Mammography," *Townsend Letter for Doctors and Patients,* December 1994, page 1390.

6. John W. Gofman, as quoted by Burton Goldberg and the editors of *Alternative Medicine Guide to Women's Health 2* (Tiburon, CA: Future Medicine, 1998), page 66.

7. Lorraine Day, as quoted in Goldberg and the editors of *Alternative Medicine Guide to Women's Health 2,* page 86.

8. Charles B. Simone, *Breast Health* (Garden City Park, NY: Avery, 1995), page 217.

9. Joseph M. Mercola, "Hormone Replacement Causally Related to Breast Cancer," *Townsend Letter for Doctors and Patients,* August/September 1998, page 24.

10. John Lee, "Is Natural Progesterone the Missing Link in Osteoporosis Prevention and Treatment?" *Medical Hypotheses* (1991).

11. John Morgenthaler and Jonathan V. Wright, "Don't Let Your Doctor Give You Horse Urine," *Anti-Aging Newsletter,* pages 8–12.

Chapter 10: Water Drinking

1. Andrew Weil, *8 Weeks to Optimum Health* (New York: Knopf, 1997), pages 64–65.

Chapter 11: Mental Detoxing

1. Psalm 46:1, *New American Standard Bible,* marginal note.

2. Isaiah 41:10, Psalm 34:3, *New American Standard Bible.*

3. Jeff Harkins, as quoted in Carrol Johnson Shewmake, *When We Pray for Others,* pages 34, 35.

Chapter 12: Liver/Gallbladder Flushing

1. Michael Murray and Joseph Pizzorno, *Encyclopedia of Natural Medicine* (Rocklin, CA: Prima, 1991), page 78.

Chapter 13: Dental Detoxing

1. Toxic Element Research Foundation, Colorado Springs, CO, 1-800-331-2303.
2. Hal Huggins, "Dental Toxins: Your Teeth May Be Making You Sick," *Alternative Medicine Digest,* May 1998, page 51.
3. Thomas Levy, "Teeth—The Root of Most Disease?" *Extraordinary Science,* April/May/June 1994.
4. Jane Heimlich, "How to Be a Savvy Dental Patient," *Health and Healing,* April 1996, supplement, page 2.
5. Dietrich Klinghardt, "9 Steps to Detox from Mercury Fillings," *Alternative Medicine Digest,* May 1999, page 12.

Chapter 15: Soaks and Saunas

1. W. John Diamond and W. Lee Cowden with Burton Goldberg, *Definitive Guide to Cancer* (Tiburon, CA: Future Medicine, 1997), page 579.
2. Keith Block, as quoted in Diamond and Cowden with Goldberg, page 61.

Chapter 16: Rebounding

1. Bruce Fife, *The Detox Book* (Colorado Springs, CO: HealthWise, 1997), page 131.
2. Morton Walker, "Jumping for Health," *Townsend Letter for Doctors and Patients,* July 1995, page 44.
3. Fife, page 131.
4. Walker, page 44.

Chapter 18: Juice Fasting and Colon/Liver Cleansing

1. Sherry A. Rogers, *Wellness Against All Odds* (Syracuse, NY: Prestige, 1994), pages 81, 88.
2. Patrick Quillin, *Beating Cancer with Nutrition* (Tulsa, OK: Nutrition Times Press, 1994), page 106.

3. James F. Balch and Phyllis A. Balch, *Prescription for Nutritional Healing* (Garden City Park, NY: Avery, 1997), pages 545, 546.

4. Max Gerson, *A Cancer Therapy* (Bonita, CA: Gerson Institute, 1990), pages 190, 191.

5. Linda Rector Page, *Healthy Healing* (Sacramento, CA: Spilman, 1990), page 32.

6. Paavo Airola, *How to Get Well* (Sherwood, OR: Health Plus, 1996), page 215.

7. Balch and Balch, page 548.

Chapter 19: The 80/20 Diet

1. Joel Robbins, *Enzymes for Health* (cassette tape presentation), available from Vitality Unlimited, P.O. Box 322, Colonia, NJ 07067, 1-800-93-VITAL.

Chapter 20: Hormone Balancing with Natural Progesterone

1. John R. Lee, *Natural Progesterone and Women's Health* (cassette tape presentation), Astraea, Inc., Women's Health Research.

2. Ibid.

3. Joseph M. Mercola, "Hormone Replacement Causally Related to Breast Cancer," *Townsend Letter for Doctors and Patients,* August/September 1998, page 24.

4. Ibid.

5. Joseph M. Mercola, "New Information on Natural Progesterone and Cancer Prevention," *Townsend Letter for Doctors and Patients,* December 1998, page 80.

6. Ibid.

7. Ibid.

Chapter 23: Essential Oils and Aromatherapy

1. Gary Young, *An Introduction to Young Living Essential Oils and Aromatherapy* (Salt Lake City, UT: Essential Press, 1996), page 12.

2. Ibid.

3. Ibid., page 7.

Chapter 25: Magnet Therapy

1. Julian Whitaker, "A Magnetic Approach to Pain Relief," *Health and Healing,* February 1998, page 6.

2. Michael B. Schachter, as quoted in W. John Diamond and W. Lee Cowden with Burton Goldberg, *Definitive Guide to Cancer* (Tiburon, CA: Future Medicine, 1997), page 386.

3. Compilation of research findings of Albert Roy Davis, Robert O. Becker, and William H. Philpott, as summarized in American Health Service Magnetics catalog.

Chapter 26: Massage Therapy

1. American Massage Therapy Association, *Guide to Massage Therapy in America,* page 10, 1130 W. North Shore Ave., Chicago, IL 60626-4670, (312) 761-AMTA.

2. M. Hernandex-Reif, T. Field, G. Ironson, et al., as reported in Tiffany M. Field, "Massage Therapy Effects," *American Psychologist,* December 1998, page 1277. Also see M. Hernandez-Reif, T. Field, G. Ironson, S. Weiss, and M. A. Fletcher (1998), "Massage Therapy for Breast Cancer" (manuscript submitted for publication).

3. Ibid.

Chapter 27: Additional Helpful Therapies

1. Burton Goldberg Group, *Alternative Medicine* (Tiburon, CA: Future Medicine, 1993), page 275.

Chapter 31: The AMAS Blood Test

1. C. Botti, A. Martinetti, S. Nerini-Molteni, L. Ferrari, "Anti-malignin Antibody Evaluation: A Possible Challenge for Cancer Management" (Nuclear Medicine Division, National Cancer Institute, Milan, Italy), *International Journal of Biological Markers,* October/December 1997, pages 141–147.

2. Lee Cowden, *Preventing and Reversing Cancer* (tape series) (Richardson, TX: Great Health).

Chapter 32: Dark Field Microscopy

1. W. John Diamond and W. Lee Cowden with Burton Goldberg, *Definitive Guide to Cancer* (Tiburon, CA: Future Medicine, 1997), page 728.

2. Douglas Brodie, quoted in Diamond and Cowden with Goldberg, page 731.

Chapter 33: Hair, Fingernail, and Tongue Observations

1. Great Smokies Diagnostic Laboratory, *Elemental Analysis* (Asheville, NC: 1997), page 2.

2. Linda Rector-Page, *Healthy Healing* (Sacramento, CA: Spilman, 1990), page 223.

Chapter 35: Stool Observations

1. Robert Gray, *The Colon Health Handbook* (Reno, NV: Emerald, 1991), page 18.

2. National Cancer Institute, *PDQ Cancer Information Supportive Care Statement—Constipation, Impaction and Bowel Obstruction,* Bethesda, MD, September 1, 1993, page 3.

3, Michael T. Murray and Joseph E. Pizzorno, *Encyclopedia of Natural Medicine* (Rocklin, CA: Prima, 1991), page 56.

4. Ibid., page 51.

ABOUT THE AUTHOR

DAVE FRÄHM is the cofounder and director of HealthQuarters Ministries, a nonprofit organization in Colorado Springs. Coauthor of *A Cancer Battle Plan, Healthy Habits,* and *Reclaim Your Health,* he is also a frequent lecturer across the country.

LEAD A HEALTHIER LIFE WITH THESE EXCEPTIONAL BOOKS FROM JEREMY P. TARCHER/PUTNAM.

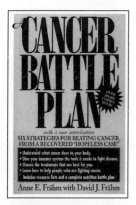

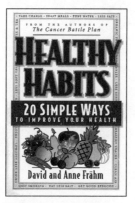

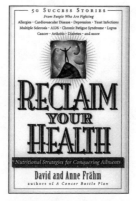

A Cancer Battle Plan: Six Strategies for Beating Cancer

An updated edition of the comprehensive nutritional battle plan that one woman used to become completely cancer free. More than 200,000 copies sold!

ISBN 0-87477-893-X
$12.95 ($18.99 CAN)

Healthy Habits: 20 Simple Ways to Improve Your Health

While most of us have only a few critical bad habits standing in the way of improved health, often our most dangerous tendencies are things we believe are good for us. Using the strategies proposed in this book, you'll learn how to replace bad habits with good ones and how to help yourself to better health.

ISBN 0-87477-918-9
$12.95 ($18.99 CAN)

Reclaim Your Health: Nutritional Strategies for Conquering Ailments

A collection of 50 success stories of people who have fought allergies, cardiovascular disease, depression, yeast infections, multiple sclerosis, AIDS, chronic fatigue syndrome, lupus, cancer, arthritis, diabetes, and other chronic illnesses and diseases using the principles of nutritional healing.

ISBN 0-87477-951-0
$12.95 ($18.99 CAN)